DATE DUE

Chasing Medical Miracles

Chasing Medical Miracles

*The Promise and Perils
of Clinical Trials*

Alex O'Meara

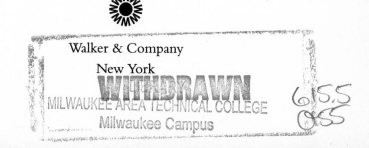

Walker & Company
New York

Published by Walker Publishing Company, Inc., New York

All papers used by Walker & Company are natural, recyclable products made
from wood grown in well-managed forests. The manufacturing processes
conform to the environmental regulations of the country of origin.

LIBRARY OF CONGRESS CATALOGING-IN-PUBLICATION DATA
HAS BEEN APPLIED FOR.

ISBN-10: 0-8027-1696-2
ISBN-13: 978-0-8027-1696-5

Visit Walker & Company's Web site at www.walkerbooks.com

First U.S. edition 2009

3 5 7 9 10 8 6 4 2

Typeset by Westchester Book Group
Printed in the United States of America by Quebecor World Fairfield

for Al Hart

CONTENTS

INTRODUCTION

WHEN I FIRST had the idea for this book I mentioned it to a friend of mine who's a doctor. "Clinical trials is a huge, *huge* area," he said. "It's important to the medical profession, to the pharmaceutical industry, to the patients. There isn't one clearinghouse, one overview about clinical trials out there. It's just huge and no one, *no one* has written about it like this."

That sounded a little over the top to me because this book was going to be about people testing drugs and medical procedures—not likely to become a movie of the week. Then I started researching clinical trials. I read articles and tracked down obscure medical journals; I went to conferences and meetings; I interviewed more doctors, subjects, nurses, patient coordinators, bioethicists, and businesspeople up and down the east coast in Washington, D.C., Philadelphia, Virginia, and New York. Then I interviewed people across the country and spoke to people around the world, in Nigeria, Thailand, and India. When that was done I went to sub-Saharan Africa because it is the perfect place to study all the complex issues associated with clinical trials. I returned from Uganda with the realization that my friend the doctor had hit the nail on the head.

There are twenty million people in the United States and fifty million people in the world enrolled in clinical trials.[1] That number has gone up 300 percent in the last ten years.[2] It is a

$24-billion-a-year industry.[3] In a word, it's huge. When did all this happen? Why did it happen? The results of clinical trials are often written about in newspapers, but how did clinical trials grow to become this cultural phenomenon with barely anyone noticing? As a reporter and as someone who had gone through a clinical trial to cure diabetes, my curiosity was piqued.

It's not to say a lot hasn't been written about clinical trials before this book. You can find hundreds if not thousands of articles, book references, and scientific papers in peer-reviewed journals on the Internet, story after story in the business sections of magazines and newspapers, Web sites listing clinical trials, and much more. But you won't find all of it in one place. It's like the four blind guys trying to describe an elephant; everyone has a piece of it but no one has put all the pieces together to describe what the beast actually is.

I asked everyone I interviewed why clinical trials were under the radar of public consciousness and discourse. Some said it was a conspiracy of big pharmaceutical corporations: that the drug companies were keeping people from being informed so they could test drugs with impunity. While such an extreme opinion is pretty nutty, that doesn't mean conspiratorial viewpoints are without merit. They signify a very real anger toward and distrust of the "medical-industrial complex" that reveals a suspicion of clinical trials.

When I asked Paul Gelsinger, whose son died in a clinical trial, why the general public seemed to know so little about them, he said, "It's very complicated. It's not something that catches people's interest. The only time it's interesting is when there's a breakthrough. And how often does that really happen? Not very often."[4]

Other people said clinical trials don't get a lot of attention because they have a freaky stigma. They are, after all, "medical experiments," dismissed in the public consciousness as a fringe medical endeavor along the lines of Frankenstein cooking up a monster in a lab. I ran across an online front-page article in the *Tucson Citizen* headlined, "Tucson's a hot spot for clinical drug trials." It talks about how Tucson is brimming with volunteers from diverse backgrounds lining up to test the latest treatments and drugs in clinical trials. They're doing it for a lot of reasons, according to the article. Some who lack health insurance volunteer because they get free medical screenings. Some do it for cold cash. Others do it because they want to help develop the next breakthrough cancer or heart drug. The article ends by admitting that even though there have been some clinical trials that have harmed people, the business of clinical trials in Tucson is nevertheless booming and shows no signs of stopping. Beneath the online article there's a space for readers to share their comments. There was only one entry from someone calling himself "Beto N" that said, "I was wondering why my neighbor has that hand growing out of his head."[5]

Clinical trials on TV and in the movies are typically portrayed as grisly undertakings or lifesaving miracles. There are dramatic examples in real life to support each view. In India, for instance, a major pharmaceutical company routinely tests potentially dangerous experimental drugs on people so impoverished and destitute they line up because the trial represents the only "health care" they'll ever receive. On the other end of the spectrum, thanks to clinical trials the survival rate for pediatric cancer in the last two decades has gone from about 20 percent to around 80 percent today.

In this book I don't advocate for or against clinical trials. There is no soapbox under my feet, and I don't take a position on whether clinical trials are good or bad. The issues surrounding medical testing are not that simple. My goal is to make the story less complicated so it can be better understood. That's important because the phenomenon of mass participation in clinical trials reveals a lot about where medical care in general is headed. Trials are the nascent form of our health-care system; they are the first stage of tomorrow's new medicines, devices, and procedures. Clinical trials hail the very future of medicine. Each success and failure—every story—is a window into the kind and quality of treatment you will either receive or be subjected to in the years to come.

I've been a reporter for more than a decade and worked for the *Baltimore Sun, Newsday,* an NBC affiliate, the City News Bureau of Chicago, the *Danbury News Times,* and many other publications in many other places, including a radio station near Mexico. I was never a medical reporter. My interest in trials began in 2004 when I signed up to take part in a clinical trial involving an experimental transplant to cure diabetes. My experience as one of only a few hundred people to go through the procedure is part of this story, and it illustrates the kind of financial, intellectual, and emotional investments made by researchers, subjects, and many others when they become part of a clinical trial.

Before I became a subject in a clinical trial I'd had type 1 diabetes for almost thirty years. A life-threatening problem with my diabetes was the key that opened the door to a clinical trial, which in turn led to a possible cure for diabetes.

Chronically uncontrolled diabetes causes complications that attack the kidneys and shut them down. It goes after the eyes and causes blindness. It wreaks havoc on circulation, destroying the heart and cutting off blood flow to the legs so that often they have to be amputated. The number of U.S. soldiers who suffered combat injuries throughout the entire Vietnam War is equal to the number of diabetics who lost their limbs to diabetes in 2005 alone.[6] Few people die of diabetes. Instead most of the 200,000 people who succumb to it each year[7] are killed by the various and brutal complications. Every day in the United States more than 4,000 people are diagnosed with diabetes, 230 diabetics get amputations, 120 diabetics start on end-stage kidney programs, and 55 diabetics go blind.[8]

I didn't suffer from any of those tragic complications. I had "hypoglycemic unawareness"—a condition where my blood sugar, instead of staying chronically high, would plunge dangerously low and I wouldn't be aware of it. Low blood sugar, or hypoglycemia, causes seizures, coma, and in some cases even death. Blood sugar levels in a nondiabetic are between 80 and 120.[9] While my blood sugar was 1,010 when I was first diagnosed at the age of eleven, in later years, because I was an avid runner and never liked eating all that much, my blood sugar sometimes sank into the 40s, 30s, and once dropped to 16. Because the brain runs on sugar, or glucose, when a glucose reading drops that low the brain goes completely haywire. And over the years I had more than my share of hypoglycemic haywire.

One time during an English class in college I took off my glasses and tried to eat them. Then I looked over at a friend of mine and said, "Ed, I'm screwed," passed out on the floor, and went into violent seizures. Another time I woke up in a hospital with a chewed tongue and my body covered with rug burns after spending three days seizing on the wall-to-wall carpeting in my apartment. Such episodes were much worse on the people in my life than on me because I rarely remembered what happened.

Once, after I awoke from a coma during a particularly severe low blood sugar episode, doctors gave me a spinal tap because they were convinced I had something more exotic and serious than diabetes, like meningitis. Even as the cold, big-bored needle slipped into my spine I was thinking what condemned people probably think when the current starts flowing through the electric chair: There's got to be a way out of this. I wasn't sure whether to be relieved or disappointed later on when I found out the test showed my coma was only caused by plain old diabetes.

All told I was taken to a hospital emergency room in the back of an ambulance more than two dozen times because of low blood sugar. It was my one and only diabetic complication, but with each passing year, hypoglycemic unawareness came closer and closer to killing me. It was also the one thing that made it possible for me to get into a clinical trial, to have a shot at a cure, and to have the experience of what millions of other people go through when they are so sick and so desperate they'll volunteer to test unproven treatments in clinical trials. Like those millions of people, I experienced setbacks, triumphs, breakthroughs, heartbreaks, and benefits because of a clinical trial.

Those are the stories that are at the heart of this book and that make clinical trials not only a "huge" phenomenon but also a very big deal.

Chapter 1

ENTERING THE RISKY WORLD OF CLINICAL TRIALS

I NEVER WENT LOOKING for a clinical trial. Instead one found me when my insulin pump broke. When it happened I immediately threw myself a good and fairly sizable tantrum for a thirty-eight-year-old man because the pump delivered insulin into my body like a mechanical pancreas, keeping me alive. I called MiniMed, the company that made the pump, to see if they could fix it. They sent a technician named Celeste to my house. While working out the problems with my pump Celeste told my wife and me that doctors at the University of Virginia were looking to enroll qualified volunteers in a clinical trial to cure diabetes. The experimental procedure replaces the insulin-producing cells that have died in a diabetic's pancreas with living, healthy, insulin-producing cells. Because the cells are located in a part of the pancreas called the Isle of Langerhans, the cells are called islet (eye-let) cells.

Those islet cells are taken, or harvested, from a recently deceased organ donor and infused through a tube into a person's portal vein, which leads to the liver. The idea was that once in the liver, the islet cells would nestle in and produce insulin as if they were in a pancreas. It's an amazing idea. Even more amazing, according to Celeste, was that the protocol for the study stipulated that the subjects had to be completely free of diabetic complications except for hypoglycemic unawareness. They were looking for people like me.

I, however, wasn't looking for them. Like a man sentenced to life in prison who, in order to keep sane, stops thinking about the outside world, I never considered the possibility of a cure for diabetes. I had had the disease for almost thirty years. During that time many people told me about "cures" and about how some day scientists would solve the riddle of diabetes and set me free. I would listen politely then immediately put whatever they said out of my mind. I couldn't afford to think about a cure because if I did I might start resenting all the work I had to do each day managing my diabetes.

Every day I took two or more shots of insulin, tested my blood sugar four or five times, counted the carbs and calories for every scrap of food I ate, calibrated the impact of exercise on my blood sugar, and tried to avoid seizures and comas. I had spent twenty-seven years—almost ten thousand days—dealing successfully with that narrow and rigorous reality. I was raised through high school in extreme poverty, often going without food and sometimes even without medication. I rarely saw a doctor. That upbringing forced me to become my own doctor, in a way. By the time I was putting myself through college I was a pro at controlling my diabetes. Aside from the unfortunate glasses-eating incident, the only diabetes-related drama in college I suffered was the time my college roommate saw a syringe on my desk and thought he was rooming with a heroin addict.

After graduation I became a journalist in New York, Chicago, Washington, D.C., Hartford, and Tucson, Arizona. Then I embarked on a business career and was successful in marketing, which was what I was working at when I moved across the country from Arizona to Richmond, Virginia. Although I was a diabetic I had also run four marathons and was deliriously happy in my marriage. I was doing a good job with my life, and I wasn't looking to jeopardize the good health I had worked hard to attain, and maintain, by enrolling in some experiment. Plus, I didn't want to get let down chasing some miracle that was a remote possibility at best. I just wasn't in the market for a cure.

My wife thought I should be. Once Celeste solved the problem with my insulin pump and left, Traci went to work convincing me to at least call the University of Virginia and ask about the trial. "What harm could it do?" she asked. A lot, I thought. The idea of putting insulin-producing cells from a dead person's pancreas into my liver, then expecting the cells to work, sounded too much like science fiction and not enough like science. She was unrelentingly positive, however, so I said I would call and find out more about the trial.

A few days later I spoke to Winsor, the patient coordinator for the clinical trial at UVA. She said she had received inquiries from people across the country seeking to enroll and that there was a backlog of people who had yet to go through the rigorous initial screening. Only one patient had gone far enough along in the trial to be on the list to receive a transplant.

She explained that the procedure originated in Edmonton, Alberta, Canada. More than three hundred people in Canada and the United States had so far received the transplant and, although it was early in a Phase I clinical trial, the success rate was promising. She said that 20 percent of the subjects had stopped taking insulin entirely. And 50 percent had significantly reduced their insulin. This *was* promising. It meant it wasn't some quack cure.

If I wanted to be considered for the study, Winsor said, I should send her my medical records confirming I had hypoglycemic unawareness. Then I would have to undergo a slew of tests, at my own expense, to demonstrate that I met the protocol criteria for the study. They were tests that I routinely had done anyway as part of my standard health-care regime. They included an eye exam for retinopathy, a degeneration of blood vessels in the eye that causes blindness; blood tests for tissue typing, cholesterol levels, and to measure the amount of protein in my urine, which was an early indicator of kidney failure; an EKG; a dental exam; and a chest x-ray.

If the results of those tests were in acceptable ranges I would stay at the University of Virginia Medical Center for an overnight evaluation where they would run more definitive tests. If I passed the evaluation, my name would be added to the national waiting list for a pancreas from a deceased donor to be used for the islet cell transplant. Once a donor match was found, I would be infused with the islet cells and placed on antirejection drugs to suppress my immune system, just like any other transplant patient. She said I would have to take the immunosuppressants for the rest of my life. Even though it sounded daunting, I was intrigued. Winsor said she would send me details about the tests and the formal protocol for the study.

That night I had second thoughts. I told Traci that the whole thing seemed like a long, involved process and that she shouldn't get too excited because I might not pass all the tests. Besides, I said, the tests would probably be really expensive. With Traci in grad school and money tight, they might be more than we could afford. Traci said we had great health insurance through my job and the tests might be covered. She said I should at least find out. Once I did, and if they were affordable, I should get the tests done and go from there. "What harm could it do?" she said. I said I would look into getting the tests.

Sometimes subjects have to take on a level of financial commitment in their clinical trial. I had paid for the cost of the initial tests but they were tests I would have had anyway as part of taking care of my diabetes, so that wasn't a burden. I was also told I would have to pay for the lifelong antirejection drugs after the transplant and that those could run me hundreds of dollars a month if they weren't covered by my insurance. I was fine with those financial possibilities.

It turned out we had exceptional insurance. I spent the next six weeks going around Richmond visiting various doctors, getting numerous tests, and sending the results to Winsor at UVA. Every doctor and nurse I told about the clinical trial was thoroughly impressed with the technology and creativity of the procedure and with the cutting-edge medicine being performed at UVA. Some, like my general care physician, said they were even impressed with me for having the courage to pursue this. I thought that was funny. If I passed the evaluation, I wouldn't be doing much. The team at UVA would be doing most of the work. But the sentiment pumped me up. It made me think I was part of something unique. For the first time, I had the idea that a cure was not only possible, it might be possible for me. Then, with only the chest x-ray needed to complete my round of tests, everything came to a screeching halt.

Winsor called to tell me there was a change in the funding for the clinical trial. A private donor whose two children had diabetes significantly funded the study. It was his desire to help eradicate the disease. However, it apparently was not his wish at that time to pay for every aspect of accomplishing this extremely expensive goal. I was told I might need to come up with as much as ten thousand dollars for post-transplant infusions of antirejection medication. On an outpatient basis I would receive an IV of immunosuppressive drugs, and each of those sessions cost two thousand dollars. All told, I might require up to five transfusions after the transplant.

I didn't have a spare ten thousand dollars, and I didn't expect to be laying my eyes or hands on that kind of money anytime soon. I told Winsor I would call her back.

Traci and I discussed it. We talked about getting loans. We

talked about Traci delaying grad school and working. I suggested we could sell some things, like perhaps our cars. In the end we admitted that even if we were able to scrape up ten thousand dollars, it was a lot to invest in an experimental treatment that might not even work. I explained all this to Winsor. She said it was understandable but that I should have the chest x-ray taken so at least all the prescreening tests would be completed in case things eventually ended up moving forward. She would send me the consent form to study so I could become familiar with it. Things might change, she said. Grant money might come through. She would let me know.

I got the chest x-ray. Then I went hunting for another clinical trial also doing islet cell transplants that might not be as cost prohibitive. It turned out there were hundreds of people already in line at a few other hospitals conducting clinical trials in order to establish their own islet cell transplant capability. The few hospitals that were recruiting subjects, however, were for me too far away from Richmond to be practical. It became obvious that the trial at UVA, a long shot to be successful even if I received the transplant, was one of those once-in-a-lifetime opportunities. It was a chance I came close to, but one that I missed. After a week trying to locate an alternative to UVA, I hit a wall. I would not be a subject in a clinical trial attempting to cure diabetes. It was a letdown. Then it got worse.

The chest x-ray revealed a lump in the lower lobe of my right lung. It was 1.5 centimeters. The word that hit hardest was the one my doctor didn't say: "Cancer." That word, even though it was not uttered, sucked every thought out of my head. Sure, diabetes is a serious, life-threatening disease. It's a top-ten killer. Cancer, though, is a step up. That's a destroyer.

I was referred to a pulmonologist. I asked him if my past history of smoking might have given me cancer. He said it was too early to even start down that road. He said I should get a CT scan and an MRI. On the way out of his office he gave me a pat on the shoulder and said not to worry.

Those tests, and others, didn't clearly define what was going on with the nodule. The pulmonologist said the best thing was to take more images of the lump in six months to see if it grew or changed. If not, then his initial impression that it was benign would stand. If it was benign then we would just keep an eye on it with tests every two years or so to make sure it stayed that way. I left his office comforted by the results but bothered to be walking away with what looked like yet another chronic condition.

A week later I celebrated my thirty-ninth birthday. I took stock. I hadn't been thinking about the clinical trial for days. As far as I was concerned, it was in the past. My next "cancer" checkup was a while off so that got shoved to the back of my mind. It was the first time in months I didn't have a test to schedule, go to, or go through. I went to my job as a communications specialist at Capital One. I spent some time writing a proposal and editing the first chapters for a book my agent was hopeful about. I also started rewriting a novel so I could send out chapters to friends for feedback. I went for a run and thought about running my third New York City Marathon in November. (I was forced to stop when I popped a chunk of cartilage out from the underside of my right knee and had to settle for limping through a half marathon before getting arthroscopic knee surgery.) Some weeks went by. I relaxed. Then in late October the phone rang. It was Winsor. Funding for the postoperative immunosuppression had come through. The clinical trial was back on.

Winsor made sure I had studied the consent form, then asked if I could come in for an overnight evaluation. She said I was their most promising candidate. They wanted to get moving as soon as possible. How does early November sound? she asked.

Traci asked if she should be there for the evaluation. By that time I was an old hand at being in hospitals, whether for tests or disasters. I told her it would probably be best if she stayed home and dealt with school.

On a crisp early November day in 2004 I drove an hour to Charlottesville from Richmond and rode the elevator to the General Clinical Research Center (GCRC) on the eighth floor of the UVA Medical Center. I walked down a plushly carpeted hallway to the nurses' station where I found four nurses—three brunettes and one blonde. They all smiled at me.

I said hello and they greeted me warmly, like I was an old friend or a VIP.

A doctor walked up and asked, "Who do we have here?"

"This is Mr. O'Meara," one nurse said. "Our transplant candidate."

"Excellent!" he said beaming. "Excellent. Welcome."

I'd been in hospitals in five states and I'd never been treated like this. It was like I was being greeted at an airport courtesy lounge in Japan.

One nurse, who introduced herself as Emelita, led me to my room.

The walls of the hallway were oak paneled, and instead of the standard hospital interrogation-style fluorescent lights the place was illuminated by muted, soft recessed lighting. The deep carpeting and the wood muffled the sounds of voices and hospital machinery until it became a soothing background hum.

Where was the linoleum? What about the institutional green hospital walls? Where were the harsh white lights that gave you an instant headache? Where was the expert, tough, and taciturn staff? Were these people for real?

Once in my room I put my bag on the bed by the window. I had a gorgeous view of the UVA campus. I could see the University of Virginia Rotunda designed by Thomas Jefferson, and the east wing of the medical center.

I changed into shorts and a T-shirt, sat on the edge of the bed, and thought about what might happen over the next two days. I imagined undergoing a barrage of tests. Nurses would draw and centrifuge my blood. They would collect my fluids and measure them in test tubes. Numbers, reports, graphs, trends, and microgram comparisons of what happened in my body would be generated and evaluated by doctors. Information about me would be noted and debated by medical experts to see if I was a good candidate for a risky transplant that could cure diabetes.

I sat there thinking about everything that would be coming up and it suddenly freaked me out. Was I worthy of all this attention and effort? The cost of the transplant alone had to be staggering, and I wouldn't be paying a dime for it. While I was very healthy, my diabetic lifestyle hadn't been exemplary. I had downed my share of beer and pizza. Did those transgressions reveal a dark flaw in my character that made me a less-than-perfect specimen for scientific study?

Later I discovered that these are normal thoughts for some potential "guinea pigs."

A nurse came in and checked my height, weight, blood pressure, and temperature. A few minutes later, Winsor came in to brief me. I had never met her. She was tall, attractive, blithely cool, and very focused. We got right to it.

Once again she reviewed the basics of the clinical trial, the immunosuppression, and the procedure and reminded me that moving on to the transplant was contingent upon me passing the evaluation in the next two days.

The one thing giving Kenneth Brayman, M.D., the lead doctor for the clinical trial, great pause was the lump in my lung. I understood completely. He didn't want to go through curing my diabetes only to have me keel over dead from lung cancer a few years down the road. Winsor said he was actually worried that the course of immunosuppression could harm me if the nodule were bacterial or fungal. She warned me that the lump could potentially be a stumbling block to my final acceptance into the trial.

Winsor asked if I had any questions. I didn't. Then she reviewed what would actually happen over the next two days, compared to what I imagined might happen during the evaluation. My blood would be drawn six times in two days to test for viruses, red and white cell counts, fat, hemoglobin A1c (to test my blood sugar level over the last three months), liver function, C-peptide, thyroid function, reactive antibodies, and clotting. Urine tests would screen for creatinine, protein, and microalbumin to assess my kidney function. I would have another chest x-ray, a liver and stomach ultrasound, an EKG, an eye exam, a tuberculosis test, and a psychosocial/psychological evaluation. I would also have tissue-typing tests to determine my cell characteristics in order to match me up with the donor cells.

Toward the end of my stay, I would take a glucose tolerance test. This would tell the team whether or not my own islet cells were producing any insulin at all. As part of the test, I would forgo insulin that morning and drink a sweet and icky solution that would send my blood sugar through the roof. They would hit me with six more blood draws, one every thirty minutes for three hours to see exactly how high my blood sugar went as a way of measuring whether I had any insulin-producing activity at all.

Before leaving the hospital the next day, I would be hooked up to a glucose monitor to wear for three days. It would record my blood sugar level every five minutes. A needle, inserted under the skin on my hip, was attached to a two-foot wire connected to a monitor the size of my hand. They would give me a little plastic bag to put the monitor in and hang around my neck whenever I took a shower.

"How does all that sound?" Winsor asked.

"Sounds great," I said. "Sounds like a party. Let's go."

Before we got going—before a single test was conducted—Winsor asked if I had any questions about the consent form. It was a twenty-two-page document so there were a few things to discuss. Afterward, I signed it and handed it to Winsor, who made me a copy. Now we were ready to move forward.

A few minutes after Winsor left, Dr. Brayman walked in.

His name tag said Professor, and I remembered that I was at a teaching hospital. That was reassuring. His appearance was comforting. He had a receding hairline, wore round glasses, and carried an open can of Diet Coke in one of his lab coat pockets.

He told me the trial and the transplant would closely follow the original protocol for islet cell transplants developed at the University of Edmonton in Alberta, Canada. It would only differ by including steroids at the time of infusion.

As he spoke I noticed that, even to a born New Yorker like me, Dr. Brayman came off as an intense guy.

He told me only about three hundred people in the world had received islet transplants.

"How many at UVA?" I asked.

"One," he said.

"Excuse me? Did you say 'One'?"

"Yes."

I asked a few more questions and received answers like "That's what we'll find out," and "That's what we're hoping for, but we'll have to see."

That was the moment when it finally sunk in. I was a *test* subject. I was the monkey in the space capsule. This transplant was *experimental*. I was a guinea pig. I had donated my body to science and I wasn't even dead.

I was part of a clinical trial, and like every single clinical trial before or since, there were no guarantees. They had told me all this. I even read and signed a twenty-two-page document attesting to it. This though was the first time it was coming through loud and clear.

The trial up until now had been like taking a trip to Disney World. Before your plane takes off they tell you in detail what to do if it becomes a fireball of screaming death and dives nose first into the ground. But you don't hear that part. You're too busy thinking about shaking hands with Goofy.

Later that day Susan Kirk, M.D., an endocrinologist who specializes in diabetes care, visited me. She had type 1 diabetes and had lived with it for almost thirty years. She was smart and very kind. Because she was a diabetic compadre, I asked if she would consider getting an islet cell transplant. No, she said, she wouldn't.

"But I don't have hypoglycemic unawareness, like you do," she said. "I might consider it in the future, once the procedure is perfected."

On the second day of the evaluation, at six thirty in the morning, they started the glucose tolerance test. The test sent my blood sugar soaring, exactly as it was meant to. They drew blood every half hour for three hours, just like they said they would. Afterward, Winsor jabbed my hip with a needle and hooked me up to the glucose monitor. Then, because she was supposed to, she officially asked me whether I wanted to go through with the clinical trial. I said yes. She said she would be in touch about what happened next. I took my morning shot of insulin, waited at the hospital until my blood sugar went back to normal range, got my parking validated, and went on my way.

With time to think during the drive home I asked myself, What the hell am I getting myself into? Do I want to go through with this?

I set aside the remote possibility of a cure. They wouldn't actually be curing me at this point anyway. If I went on to the next phase, it was only for an experimental procedure with long odds.

Lottery odds. Worse than lottery odds. It was a lottery that, even if I won, might not pay out. And at this point I was only being allowed to get in line to see if I could even buy a ticket. Despite that, there was something compelling and exciting about the prospect of following this through to the end. I decided right then that I wanted to see, wanted to find out, what was possible.

Three weeks later I received a letter saying I had been accepted for candidacy into the clinical trial. I was placed on the Pancreas Islet Cell Transplant waiting list with restrictions. There were three catches. Two of them were no big deal. Per the protocol for the study, I needed to start seeing an endocrinologist on a regular basis. I also needed to repeat a blood test for tissue typing. The third restriction was more problematic. I needed to have more tests on the nodule in my lung. If it was anything other than a benign mass, I was out of the clinical trial and my hope for a cure was over. I had no idea the extraordinary lengths I would go to in order to make sure that didn't happen.

Chapter 2

THE RIGHT AND WRONG
OF CLINICAL TRIALS

TWO WORDS. The most significant ethical issue in clinical trials can be summed up in two words. That's quite an accomplishment considering how flexible and slippery the concept of right and wrong has remained throughout the thousands of years since researchers and scientists began testing drugs and treatments on people.[1] The cast of characters who shaped the ethics of clinical trials, such as they stand today, includes Greek philosophers, snake-oil salesmen, the Nazis, government committees, geniuses, Nobel Prize winners, miracle workers, racist doctors, stressed-out parents, poor, illiterate Southern blacks, dedicated humanitarians, thousands of brave souls, and some very unlucky subjects. Given that complicated lineage, it's a wonder that the major ethical issue in clinical trials can be summed up at all, never mind in just two words.

Clinical trials yield miraculous treatment options: everything from citrus fruit to treat scurvy to heart, liver, kidney, pancreas, and other lifesaving transplants. They have produced treatments and drugs for thousands of diseases and conditions such as cancer, HIV/AIDS, lupus, syphilis, diabetes, tuberculosis, heart disease, smallpox, and more. Some clinical trials study profound ailments, such as pediatric cancer. Others research the trivial. One clinical trial studied whether breathing through just one nostril was more calming than breathing through both, concluding that such a practice "could have a marked activating effect or relaxing effect on the sympathetic nervous system."[2]

Today, because of clinical trials, life-prolonging devices such as kidney stents, asthma inhalers, heart valves, insulin pumps, pacemakers, and even entire artificial hearts are available to those who can benefit from them. Making questionable and controversial ethical decisions is part of how these amazing triumphs took place. The ways in which substantial ethical roadblocks were ignored, negotiated, and leveled raises questions about whether the benefits reaped are really worth the atrocities committed and the horror endured and about whether such questionable practices remain in the past.

Terrible things happen in clinical trials because they are the most dangerous part of medical discovery. And medical discovery is not an exact science. It seems to have more in common with improvisational performance art than it does with science. That's because medical discovery is complex and nuanced. It's never a scientist in a lab adding a substance to a test tube then shouting "Eureka!" Very little in medical research, of which clinical trials are only the final phase, goes according to plan. The process requires equal parts creativity, intuition, tenacity, scientific skill, and plain old dumb luck.

An example of how most medical breakthroughs come about can be found in the century-long quest to bring a cervical cancer vaccine to the clinical trial phase of development. The path involved decades of mistakes, breakthroughs, and false leads—plus the participation of cows, nuns, prostitutes, and rabbits. In 1842 an Italian doctor in Florence noticed that cervical cancer struck married woman and prostitutes, while nuns appeared unaffected by the condition, which he attributed to the nuns' corsets being too tight.

That was just the first in a long, strange list of conclusions. Over the years, doctors drew causal links between cervical cancer and circumcision, herpes, salt, sexual abstinence, and the avoidance of bacon by Jewish women.

In the 1930s Richard Shope, M.D., a doctor at Rockefeller University in New York, became aware that some wild rabbits had "horns." These protrusions were actually warts that appeared similar to those associated with cervical cancer. Curious about them, the doctor ran tests and discovered, for the first time, that a virus caused the warts.

Because human warts contain very little virus from which to create a vaccine, in the 1980s William Bonnez, M.D., at the University of Rochester tried to extract the virus from dairy cows, which apparently grow warts the size of avocados. Dr. Bonnez also set out to formulate a human blood test for the virus. For that, he needed a control group of women who had never had sex. The Sisters of St. Joseph in Rochester, New York, answered extensive questions about their sexual histories (or lack thereof), gave blood samples, and added a lot of valuable information to development of a vaccine.

"People were snickering," Dr. Bonnez said. "Ha-ha, nuns, no sex. But having a control group of fifty subjects—that led me to realize the bovine approach was wrong."

Further development and refinement of the theory, followed by legal wrangling between two giant pharmaceutical companies for thirteen years, finally produced a vaccine. Afterward, the vaccine was further refined and tested in clinical trials before the U.S. Food and Drug Administration (FDA) approved it in 2006 for use by the general public.[3]

It's practically impossible to regulate and even manage a process as confounding as that. To impose rigid ethical guidelines in an inherently intuitive process like medical discovery could strangle the process until it becomes so stifled that important discoveries remain unexplored. The problem, though, is that clinical trials are the one part of medical discovery where human lives are put directly at risk. Also, as history amply demonstrates, in the absence of guidelines and agreed-upon definitions of what is ethical and not ethical, subjects in clinical trials get trampled in the blind pursuit of trying to apply medical breakthroughs.

One of the first clinical trials is mentioned in the Old Testament. In 650 BCE, King Nebuchadnezzar II observed that the prophet Daniel, who ate bread and drank water, looked healthier than his subjects, who ate meat and drank wine. Nebuchadnezzar suspected Daniel's diet of bread and water could be why he enjoyed superior overall health. To find out, he switched his subjects to Daniel's regime. They became healthy and he instituted a diet change.[4] And as simply as that, voilà, successful clinical trial.

In 1747 James Lind, a Scottish doctor serving aboard HMS *Salisbury*, conducted a clinical trial to identify the definitive cure for scurvy. The condition, which caused loose teeth, hemorrhaging, and bleeding gums, was a widespread health problem for men serving aboard ships. Instead of trying out possible cures one at a time on groups of men until he hit upon one that worked, he tried something new. He got together a group of twelve men who were suffering from scurvy. In groups of two he gave them several different possible cures, including seawater; vinegar; a vile cocktail of garlic, horseradish, and mustard; and, for the last lucky two, oranges and lemons. While the powers of citrus had long been anecdotally known to help treat scurvy, thanks to Lind it was absolutely proven to be the one sure remedy and was adopted as the standard treatment for the condition. What Lind also discovered was how to conduct a more efficient study by making his test a parallel trial. By giving one group—the control group—citrus and comparing the results against the groups who took treatments that were suspected of not working, he invented the placebo trial. For more than 150 years researchers voluntarily adopted placebos and control groups as a standard guideline for conducting clinical trials.[5]

In the twentieth century, snake-oil salesmen, who were audaciously labeling and selling any concoction as "healthful" even though it might only be tap water, alcohol, or some truly harmful potion, inadvertently contributed to formalizing regulations for clinical trials. To stem the growing flood of false claims made for such "medicines," in 1906 Congress passed the Pure Food and Drug Act, a law that made selling mislabeled food and drugs across state lines a crime. Drug Laboratory, a federal department that today is the Center for Drug Evaluation and Research (CDER), enforced the new law. The Drug Laboratory back then was part of the Bureau of Chemistry, or what is known today as the FDA.[6]

In 1910 it was discovered that the Pure Food and Drug Act had a loophole when the Bureau of Chemistry impounded something called Johnson's Mild Combination Treatment for Cancer. It may have been too mild because it had no therapeutic benefits at all. The government took Johnson's to court to stop them from selling the cancer treatment. The judge, surprisingly, sided with the makers of Johnson's Mild Combination and said the law didn't cover claims of effectiveness of "medicines." Congress shut that loophole two years later by adding the Sherley Amendment to the act.[7] The amendment effectively forced companies selling medicines to conduct clinical trials to prove the claims they put on their labels. If the companies showed in the trials that their panaceas worked, they were allowed to lawfully make the claim on the label.[8]

These government regulations were the first of many efforts to create agreed-upon and enforceable guidelines regulating the processes ensuring that people are receiving safe and properly tested drugs and medical treatments. They were also the first of many such guidelines and laws that created the currently complicated procedures for conducting clinical trials. "Organized clinical research is a creature of the second half of the twentieth century," according to Dr. Paul Appelbaum, a bioethicist at the New York Psychiatric Institute and Hospital, which is affiliated with Columbia University. "Historically, clinical research in general, not just clinical trials, began with a very patchwork set of ethical principles underlying it. For many reasons, some accurate and others not, that reputation persists."[9]

From the mid-twentieth century onward, researchers on their own have employed new methods or revised old ones to make clinical trials more effective. To ensure they also remain safe, governments and other groups passed laws and regulations defining what is ethical and not ethical in clinical trials. But the regulations and the actions taken by researchers on their own are usually reactive. They address previous atrocities in medical experimentation, but the regulations and practices rarely, if ever, prevent the future mistreatment of subjects. The hundreds of rules have had the unexpected consequence of increasing the involvement of nonmedical groups and people, such as lawyers, in clinical testing, which has made clinical trials very complex and controversial.

Early in the twentieth century, for example, randomization was introduced to clinical trials and quickly became recognized as the most significant improvement in helping to generate more accurate data since the placebo. Subjects are divided into two groups, as before, with one receiving the treatment being tested and the other being given a placebo. But to prevent biased results, the tests are blinded. They are either single-blinded, which means that the subjects don't know whether they're getting the placebo or the treatment, or they're double-blinded, which means that the subjects *and* the researchers conducting the study don't know whether the treatment or the placebo is being administered. Randomization helps ensure that subjects won't report feeling better because they think they're being treated—the so-called placebo effect. It also prevents researchers from skewing the results in favor of whatever they're testing because they don't know which subjects are getting the treatment and which are not.[10]

While it was a major step forward in improving clinical trials, the randomization method didn't make trials much safer. That would require new laws, which were passed only after a horrific trial testing a drug called Elixir Sulfanilamide killed more than one hundred people in 1937. The drug had been successfully tested and used for years, as a powder and as a pill, to treat streptococcal infections, which cause strep throat, among other ailments. Then one day a salesman for the manufacturer S. E. Massengill Company, in Bristol, Tennessee, asked the lab to make the drug into a liquid, because that's how Southern customers would prefer to take it. Raspberry flavoring was added, the drug was control-tested in the lab to ensure flavor and appearance, and 240 gallons of the stuff was shipped across the country. It was not, however, tested on people. The additive that turned the drug to a liquid was diethylene glycol, a chief ingredient in antifreeze.[11]

The entire staff of more than two hundred inspectors who at the time worked for the FDA fanned out across the country and successfully recovered most of the drug that had been shipped. One indirect fatality from the incident was Harold Watkins, the chemist who developed the liquid form of the drug. Overcome with remorse, Watkins committed suicide when he learned what had happened. But the owner of the company, Samuel Evans Massengill, M.D., said, "My chemists and I deeply regret the fatal results, but there was no error in the manufacture of the product. We have been supplying a legitimate professional demand and not once could have foreseen the unlooked-for results. I do not feel that there was any responsibility on our part."[12] Massengill was correct. The company technically did nothing wrong because in 1937 it wasn't illegal to sell untested drugs even if they were toxic. No law regulating clinical testing for safety had been enacted. In 1938 Congress rectified that oversight and strengthened the Pure Food and Drug Act by passing the Food, Drug, and Cosmetic Act, which still forms the basis for the FDA's oversight of drugs and consumer products.

That act was further refined in 1941 when the Insulin Amendment was added to the Food, Drug, and Cosmetic Act. The amendment required that insulin should be tested for "purity, strength, quality, and identity before marketing." The amendment was applicable to other drugs that needed approval from the FDA as well. That same year the FDA also required prescription labeling for new drugs.[13] This legislation can be considered the tipping point that led to the eventual creation of the $24 billion-a-year clinical trials industry that is in place today.

The pattern in the United States of responding to atrocities in clinical trials with new regulations to guide ethical behavior was about to be repeated on a global scale. Brutal experiments conducted on a systematic basis led, paradoxically, to the first worldwide agreement on the proper treatment of subjects in clinical trials when, between 1939 and 1945, Nazi Germany's medical establishment conducted at least seventy experiments on more than seventy thousand people at Birkenau, Dachau, Auschwitz, and other concentration camps. Doctors and scientists ran tests to gather information about genetic engineering, new drugs, the effects of sterilization, protection of military personnel, and supposed cures for injury, illness, and disease. Jews, Gypsies, Poles, Soviet prisoners of war, mentally disabled people, children of all races, and others were subjected to torturous experimentation—many forced into serving as test subjects until the experiments killed them. Afterward they were often dissected and studied further.[14]

Nazis would place a person in a tank of cold water or put them outside in the snow to determine the exact temperature at which they would freeze to death. Sometimes, when the freezing person was near death, doctors would pump hot water into the person's rectum to see how long it would take to revive them. Doctors switched limbs and organs on twin children. They operated on people without anesthesia. To replicate combat conditions they shot subjects with poison bullets then rubbed wood, gravel, and glass into the wounds to determine the best ways to treat wounded German soldiers in the field.[15]

(Ironically, in 1931 a set of *Reichtlinein*, or regulations, had been passed in Germany that said subjects in clinical trials must give consent in "a clear and undebatable manner."[16] The regulations obviously were ignored during World War II.)

The Nazi experiments were not only inhumane. They were also bad science. Nazi doctors routinely took credit for the work they forced upon prisoner-doctors. Research methods, records, and results were rarely verified or confirmed, and there was little to no independent oversight or regulation of experiments. Doctors frequently ran tests based on nothing more than personal whim.

Josef Mengele, M.D., experimented extensively on twins at Auschwitz. The topic of twins fascinated him because he thought twins might hold the key to developing a system of race purification. Mengele became convinced that two twin boys he was experimenting on had tuberculosis, even though exhaustive tests did not reveal the condition. Mengele left a meeting where prisoner-doctors assured him the boys did not have tuberculosis. Mengele shot the two boys in the neck and before their bodies cooled, dissected them and examined every organ himself. He returned an hour later and said, "You were right. There was nothing."[17]

"Mengele was obviously psychotic," says Ken Faulkner, a chaplain, bioethicist, and director of clinical services at the Medical College of Virginia. "He was somebody with no conscience. He was a sociopath with a physician's training."[18]

The reaction to the Nazi experiments resulted in the creation of the most important document guiding the ethics of clinical trials in the history of medical research to date.[19] The Nuremberg Medical Trial, charging twenty-three Nazi doctors with experimenting on subjects without their consent or knowledge, convened on December 9, 1946.[20] Two years later, in 1948, the Nuremberg Code was ratified. The Code was the first international statement that specified how researchers and doctors should treat subjects. Previously, the Hippocratic oath—"First do no harm"—was the primary ethical guide for researchers conducting clinical trials.

The judges at the Nuremberg Medical Trial wanted something stronger, a document devoted solely to the treatment of subjects. Although the ten articles of the code were never made law by any country and it does not carry the force of law, the code remains important because it stipulates that subjects have to give voluntary consent to participate in trials, that they have to be informed of the risks, and that the risks to the subject have to equal the potential benefit to the subject and society. Also importantly, two articles of the code empower subjects so they can protect themselves and not have to rely solely on the actions of researchers and physicians to provide protection. The first article says, "The voluntary consent of the human subject is absolutely essential." The ninth article says, "During the course of the experiment the human subject should be at liberty to bring the experiment to an end if he has reached the physical or mental state where continuation of the experiment seems to him to be impossible."[21]

The Nuremberg Code prompted governments in the United States and around the world to look at clinical trials and take steps to protect the subjects who were enrolled in them. As a result, the World Health Organization (WHO), the FDA, the National Institutes of Health (NIH), and other organizations today regulate clinical trials much more stringently.[22]

"I think the history of Nuremberg in particular is a complicated one in terms of the impact that it had on American research," Appelbaum says. "It raises issues about patient consent, coercion and what that constitutes, and many other topics that we continue to address."[23]

Whether or not to apply the results of Nazi experiments to patient care is a thorny issue that continues to be debated by medical professionals. Several times serious researchers have proposed gathering the information from experiments carried out in concentration camps so it can be considered for serious scientific debate and potential application. The director of the Hypothermia Laboratory at the University of Minnesota in Duluth sought to have data from Nazi experiments on freezing then rewarming people published in the *New England Journal of Medicine*. The author's argument was that because of the extremity of the Nazi experiments, the data today would otherwise be unobtainable and, therefore, has scientific value. The article was flatly rejected because of how the data for the "trial" was collected.[24]

In 1989 the U.S. Environmental Protection Agency studied phosgene gas, used in manufacturing plastics and pesticides, to see if it should be regulated as a potentially life-threatening pollutant. Exposure to even small concentrations of the gas was suspected to attack lung enzymes, causing fluid buildup and potentially killing people who lived in areas where plastics and pesticides are manufactured. To answer the question about how to proceed with regulation, researchers sifted through existing clinical trials to find any previous experiments with phosgene gas that were performed on human subjects. They came up with nothing. They were resigned to settling for less accurate and less reliable animal testing when a consulting firm working for the EPA unearthed phosgene gas testing that had been conducted by Nazi researchers. The tests had killed four French prisoners in World War II. The EPA sought to reject the Nazi data because they didn't think it was reliable. When the consultant dug in and proved the data would be useful, twenty-two EPA scientists wrote a letter objecting to using the data because it originated with the Nazis. The EPA's chief administrator, Lee Thomas, made the final decision not to use the data because it might expose the agency to serious criticism.

Baruch Cohen, writing on the topic in the publication *Jewish Law*, said Thomas's decision was a "knee jerk reaction" that was "typical . . . but unprofessional."[25] Thousands of U.S. citizens at the time were living near manufacturing plants emitting phosgene gas. Getting the most accurate picture of how the gas might harm them, Cohen argued, could save lives.[26]

Scholars, however, are finding that references to Nazi research, and even the work of former doctors who served in Hitler's SS, are quietly creeping into established medical journals.[27] They are showing up because the medical community lacks clear-cut ethical guidelines providing direction on how to treat the results.

Nazi Germany didn't have a monopoly on conducting unethical and deadly clinical trials. The infamous Tuskegee study was sponsored by the United States government and conducted in Macon County, Alabama, with the cooperation of researchers from the Tuskegee Institute. The "Tuskegee Study of Untreated Syphilis in the Negro Male," as it was officially called, was designed to find out if syphilis affected black people and white people differently.[28] Doctors from the United States Public Health Service (PHS) studied 201 African-American men who did not have syphilis and 399 others who did without ever telling the subjects about their real illness, without getting their consent, and without offering lifesaving treatment to the men when such treatment became available. When it started, researchers thought the study would last six months. It ended up lasting from 1932 to 1972.[29]

Researchers in the clinical trial tracked men with syphilis until they died from the untreated condition then collected data by autopsy. Death from untreated syphilis in the late, or tertiary stage, is excruciating and brutal. Syphilis usually attacks the heart and central nervous system and even spreads to the brain and spinal cord, which causes many victims to walk with a "stumbling gait" or renders them permanently paralyzed, insane, blind, and deaf.[30]

Most of the sharecroppers and farmhands who took part in the study were poor and illiterate, and all of them were black. Many of the men were recruited from farms after doctors convinced farm owners they should enroll their workers in the study. The subjects were directly enticed into the study with promises of free overall medical care, transportation to and from the clinic where they were examined, a hot meal when they went to be examined, and the promise of a fifty-dollar burial stipend so their families wouldn't be overburdened by the expense of their deaths.[31] The men were grateful to receive free medical treatment for what doctors told them was "bad blood," a local euphemism for a wide variety of sicknesses, and they appreciated having burial insurance.[32]

The Nuremberg Code wasn't the only set of guidelines for ethical treatment in research ignored by researchers conducting the Tuskegee study. In 1964 the World Health Organization passed the Helsinki Declaration specifically guiding the actions of doctors involved in clinical research.[33] The declaration further refines what is stated in the Nuremberg Code about what should be considered ethical and unethical in clinical trials. It reiterates that subjects give informed consent in trials. It says an independent board should review the procedures of trials; that lab and animal testing should precede testing on humans; that the risk in the trial should not exceed the benefits of the trial; and that trials should be conducted by scientifically and/or medically qualified experts.[34]

On the last point, the Tuskegee study was completely in compliance. Every one of the doctors taking part in the study was eminently qualified and their actions were overseen by the PHS, a federal agency designated to protect the health of U.S. citizens. That the government, through the PHS, sponsored the study was to many the most chilling aspect of the Tuskegee study. When it became widely reported, the editor of the *Providence Sunday Jour-*

nal reflected popular opinion at the time by saying he was astounded by "the flagrant immorality of what occurred under the auspices of the United States Government."[35] Government health officials were directly involved with the smallest details of the study by the government. The surgeon general, the nation's top doctor, even issued each man a certificate of appreciation twenty-five years into the study.[36]

The Tuskegee study was widely publicized in 1972 after one of the Public Health Service staff involved in the study spoke to an Associated Press reporter. Afterward the study was shut down in the face of public outrage. The PHS has never officially apologized. It said at the time that the men were "volunteers."[37]

By the time the experiment was stopped, twenty-eight of the men were dead from untreated syphilis, one hundred died of related complications, forty wives of the men had the disease, and nineteen of their children were born with it. The most disturbing fact is that thirteen years into the study, it was discovered that penicillin probably could have cured the men.[38]

"Tuskegee fits almost all the negative characteristics of a clinical trial you can identify," Dr. Appelbaum said. "No consent. There was deception and needless harm. There wasn't even a clear scientific justification for the study to begin with."[39]

The Tuskegee study continues to impact the lives of African Americans today. One arguable legacy is that blacks continue to have a deep mistrust of the medical establishment. Neil Powe, M.D., a professor of medicine at Johns Hopkins School of Medicine in Baltimore who was involved in a 2007 study, says, "We found that minorities are 200 percent more likely to perceive harm coming from participating in research."[40] Powe says that high level of mistrust is a direct legacy of the Tuskegee study.[41] He notes the unfortunate irony that the low level of participation by blacks in clinical trials makes it difficult for researchers to study how to treat conditions affecting blacks at higher rates than whites.

Because the Tuskegee experiment was so openly racist and in-volved the U.S. government, some black Americans believe it was part of a plot to annihilate their race and that the effort continues today. Stephen Thomas, Ph.D., director of the Institute for Minority Health Research at Emory University, and Sandra Quinn, Ph.D., at the University of North Carolina at Chapel Hill linked the Tuskegee experiment directly to a belief among blacks that AIDS was a purposeful form of genocide meant to kill blacks.[42] This is not the viewpoint of fringe groups or a few loonies in the African-American community. A poll showed that nearly half of blacks asked thought AIDS was produced in a lab by the U.S. government, and 43 percent said that the government was not revealing all there was to know about the disease.[43] High-profile African Americans, including director Spike Lee and actor Will Smith, have publicly spoken about the possibility that AIDS was produced as a result of biological testing by the government.[44]

Thirty-five years after Tuskegee, bioethicist Faulkner rejects the idea that Tuskegee was an effort to kill blacks or that the re-searchers involved in Tuskegee were evil. "These [doctors] thought they were serving a higher good," he says. "They said to themselves 'We're learning all there is to know about syphilis.' Of course, it becomes hard to defend after the widespread use of penicillin be-came the definitive cure and they withheld treatment."[45] In clinical trials, researchers sometimes are more focused on the outcome of their study—or are too blinded by racism to follow the dictates of human conscience.

Another clinical trial in which some of the most vulnerable members of society were abused was conducted from 1960 to 1963 when mentally retarded children enrolled at the Willowbrook State School in New York were deliberately infected with hepati-tis. Because the children were clearly unable to give consent, some of the children's parents signed waivers to allow the procedure.

Many did so after being told their children would be admitted to the school only if they signed the consent for the trial.[46]

Doctors justified infecting the children by claiming that hepatitis was rampant at the facility anyway, and to induce the disease by injection didn't expose the children to any greater risk of acquiring it naturally. When the trial was exposed in the media there was a public outcry over what was regarded as another example of reprehensible, government-sponsored human experimentation.[47]

Since the Willowbrook study did confirm the existence of the hepatitis A and B strains, which led to greater treatment for the public, according to Dr. Appelbaum, "The scientific justification for Willowbrook . . . put us firmly on the road to developing [a] vaccine, and yet the ethical aspects of the study were highly questionable. That in itself raises issues."[48]

Willowbrook and Tuskegee hit the headlines when the public was already encountering an avalanche of bad news about clinical trials. On the heels of the Associated Press reports about Tuskegee, other news stories revealed that the U.S. Army had tested LSD on unwitting servicemen in the 1960s. And in 1961 researchers conducting the Milgram experiments at Yale purposely misled subjects to determine if they would behave cruelly if they thought they had permission from authority figures to do so. After prompting by someone the subjects believed was in charge, the subjects delivered what they thought were electric shocks strong enough to almost kill a person sitting not ten feet away from them. These disturbing revelations added to a growing, widespread suspicion about clinical trials. The first inklings that the general public might have misgivings started, paradoxically, in 1954 when millions of American citizens embraced medical research to cure a debilitating childhood disease.

The clinical trial testing the polio vaccine developed by Jonas

Salk, M.D., was the largest such study ever undertaken or completed. More than three hundred thousand clinicians, doctors, and other health-care workers inoculated 1.8 million children with the unproven vaccine. Mothers and fathers enthusiastically took their children to 215 sites across the country where over a five-week period they received three intramuscular injections of either the vaccine or a placebo. Each inoculated child was presented with a "Polio Pioneer" ID card, a piece of candy, and a "Polio Pioneer" pin as congratulations for their contribution.[49]

The test results for each subject were tabulated on IBM punch cards and examined closely to determine if the vaccine worked or not. On April 12, 1955, ten years to the day after polio-stricken president Franklin Delano Roosevelt died, news came over the radio that the vaccine was a success.[50] People were so excited by the incredible announcement of medical triumph that some leapt from their cars, causing traffic jams across the country.[51] The joy was tempered however when it was revealed that during the trial 220 children had been infected with polio and that ten of those children had died. The vaccine that caused the infections was produced at Cutter Laboratories. Very quickly Cutter was facing sixty lawsuits, and the public's skepticism about clinical trials was entrenched.[52] By the 1970s the disturbing news about clinical trials that kept coming out in the press had turned that public disillusionment and wariness of clinical trials into outright mistrust.

Several other changes taking place in society around the same time also conspired to bring about a "patient rights" movement that gave people more direct control over their health care and brought clinical research out of the shadows and into the light of public scrutiny. In the political and social fervor of the late 1960s and 1970s, groups and individuals started challenging just about every form of the status quo and "establishment" authority, from protests against the Vietnam War and for civil rights and gay rights to efforts to pass the Equal Rights Amendment and the accompanying fight for women's rights. The Supreme Court's decision on Roe v. Wade guaranteeing a woman's right to an abortion and the high court's ruling on the Karen Ann Quinlan case guaranteeing a patient's right to die drew the public's attention to the fact that the government could and did regulate what people could and could not do with their bodies. All these contributed to a greater consciousness about health care, and that led to serious examination about how health care could be improved. In this atmosphere of new medical awareness, the way clinical research was conducted came under increasing scrutiny. This fresh look caused people and groups to demand improvements and change, even though for years no one was quite sure precisely what to change.

At the same time, the development of sophisticated medical technology (CT scans, MRIs, chemotherapy, etc.) meant treatment options and medical information started coming to patients from a team of specialists, rather than from one doctor. "The doctor was no longer the guy always in control of everything," Faulkner says. "In addition, all these other people, particularly around law and ethics started gravitating toward the bedside. Philosophers, theologians, social scientists, attorneys, and others started to speak more to the moral issue of the way health care was practiced and delivered."[53]

By the 1980s the Norman Rockwell-esque portrayal of a doctor as a benevolent, primary patient caregiver was a relic. Committees, government departments, and corporations were actively involved in health care. All these elements came together, creating a significant and fundamental shift in health care that turned passive patients into medical consumers. And those consumers wanted new treatments and that meant more clinical trials.

For clinical research, the new, inclusive model of health care meant more regulations that made the tough and costly process of testing new drugs and procedures more difficult. In order to keep turning out treatments to meet the demand, sponsors of clinical trials had to become more clever in finding ways of conducting business like they did in the old days when regulations were more lax while at the same time appearing to stringently follow the new rules. A practice of sticking to the letter of the law without adhering to the spirit of the law started creeping into clinical practice.

This tendency is exemplified in how Paul Appelbaum describes the most important ethical issue in clinical trials today in just two words: therapeutic misconception. Therapeutic misconception means that researchers who recruit and conduct clinical trials will subtly, and sometimes overtly, lead subjects to believe they are receiving medical treatment when they sign up for a clinical trial even though treatment is *never* the reason for a clinical trial. While clinical trials do sometimes provide treatment, that's only a side effect of taking part in what can sometimes be a risky proposition. The purpose of any trial is to test drugs, treatments, and devices to see if and how they work. A test pilot may set a speed record while testing a new plane, but the first and main reason he's in that plane is to find out how well it flies and if it's safe. Most of the time that is not clearly communicated to clinical trial subjects. A lawyer who specializes in clinical trials says that all the cases he tries involve therapeutic misconception.[54] It's so pervasive because it's such an effective way around the rules and regulations set up to guide clinical trials. At the same time it's not against the rules per se.

In the last thirty years hundreds of regulations have been imposed with the goal of making the sometimes-arbitrary process of medical discovery more efficient and safer. Government oversight of clinical trials has increased tremendously. Patient advocacy groups, lobbyists for large pharmaceutical companies, private research organizations, internal review boards, attorneys, journalists, and— most important—the general public are all looking over the shoulders of doctors and researchers to protect the public's interests. Participation by so many interested parties has made the process of medical discovery safer, but also much more complicated.

These days, if Nebuchadnezzar were conducting a trial to get FDA approval for a drug or treatment, there's no way he would be permitted to switch a person's diet based on a hunch about what may or may not happen. The FDA is one of the major government agencies that prevents scientists from testing people with such impunity.

The agency's drug approval process is rigorous, expensive, and complex. The FDA spells out exactly how to get a new drug approved in a report called "From Test Tube to Patient." The first step is preclinical research—which, for a drug, means the manufacturer must show proof of synthesis and purification. Afterward, the drug or treatment is tested on two animals, one rodent and one nonrodent. Scientists on behalf of the manufacturer then study the data produced by the rodents/nonrodents for any signs of compromise in expected effectiveness or unexpected test results. The manufacturer makes changes to the drug in response to these findings. This process usually takes about five years. Once the animal studies have revealed how the drug is absorbed into the bloodstream, the toxicity of the drug, how the drug is broken down chemically, and a host of other effects, an institutional review board (IRB) of independent experts and regular members of the community determines whether the drug is ready to be tested on people in a clinical trial. IRBs function as a monitoring system between the hospital, university, medical school, or corporation sponsoring the trial. There are thousands of IRBs in the United States, and they actively review events throughout the trial to ensure that all internal and government regulations are being followed.

Once the IRB gives the go-ahead, clinical trials can begin. This initiates a campaign that takes between three and seven more years of heavily regulated experimentation to determine if scientists and doctors are on the right path with their new treatment or drug.

Every legitimate clinical trial is divided into four phases. Phase I tests procedures and drugs in healthy people to determine the safety, doses, and methodology. Phase II tests a small group of between twenty and three hundred people who are suffering from the affliction or condition that the procedure or drug will treat. Phase III testing opens the trial to a larger group of people, usually between three hundred and three thousand or more, to find anomalies in new populations and uncover other effects of the drug or procedure that did not show up in the smaller Phase II test sampling. Phase IV occurs after FDA approval and is designed to gather information about widespread and long-term use. During each phase government and independent agencies are supposed to review the data from the trial in painstaking detail.[55]

All institutions that conduct clinical trials then report their test results to the FDA, the Office for Human Research Protection (OHRP) at the U.S. Department of Health and Human Services (HHS), the National Institutes of Health, and a host of other local, state, and federal agencies that enforce hundreds of regulations for clinical trials.

Even the FDA says the approval process is complicated and requires "vast amounts of time and money to complete." Investor firms caution that if you're going to sink your money into pharmaceutical companies, you'd better invest in one that already has drugs approved or has them far along in the process because the up-front costs with nothing in the pipeline can cripple a growing company. Only 20 percent of drugs submitted for FDA approval are ever sold across the counter. The price tag is between $350 million and $500 million to get a single drug through clinical trials. It generally takes anywhere from ten to nineteen years to create, study, test, and approve a new drug before it shows up in your neighborhood pharmacy.

Despite such rigorous oversight, however, mistakes still happen. In September 1999 eighteen-year-old Jesse Gelsinger died not long after receiving an injection of the common cold virus at the University of Pennsylvania Institute for Human Gene Therapy as part of a study on human gene therapy. The death was a milestone in clinical trials that prompted a precedent-setting lawsuit and congressional hearings into how gene therapy clinical trials were being conducted at the time.

Gelsinger was born with a mild form of ornithine transcarbamylase (OTC) deficiency, a genetic condition in which the liver can't metabolize the protein in food, causing levels of ammonia to build up in the blood. He controlled his condition with medications and wasn't in any distress when he volunteered for the trial. After Gelsinger died it was discovered that the researchers at Penn, according to Gelsinger's father, Paul, withheld serious facts about the trial that could have spared Jesse's life.[56]

One of the doctors involved in Gelsinger's clinical trial, Dr. James Wilson, the chairman of the University of Pennsylvania Institute for Human Gene Therapy, founded and held stock in a biotech firm that provided financial backing to the institute he chaired.[57] Asked about the apparent conflict of interest, a bioethicist from the National Institutes of Health said it didn't raise any red flags because it's not uncommon for researchers in gene therapy to also have a financial interest in the companies that are developing gene therapy treatments.[58]

Four months after Gelsinger was removed from life support and died, the FDA stopped all gene therapy experiments at Penn. From a process standpoint, the FDA and Penn researchers did a miserable job of tracking and reporting adverse reactions in subjects from other gene therapy trials.[59] Officials from the NIH and the FDA testified in front of a congressional committee that they were unsure whether gene therapy experiments had caused the death of other subjects in addition to Gelsinger. Congress heard testimony that information sharing between the NIH and FDA, the two agencies that oversee gene therapy trials, was poor and that regulations were not strictly enforced. Additionally, the NIH said researchers typically ignored government rules that they had to report negative side effects from experiments involving adenovirus, the virus that was administered to Gelsinger. After Gelsinger's death it was uncovered that there were 691 side effects that should have been reported, but only 39 were.[60]

In the months after Gelsinger died the FDA and NIH took steps to institute tougher regulations and to strengthen federal oversight of gene therapy trials, work that is still going on today. Paul Gelsinger sued the University of Pennsylvania and Penn settled the lawsuit in just two weeks for an undisclosed amount without admitting any wrongdoing.

In 2001 twenty-four-year-old Ellen Roche, a healthy employee at Johns Hopkins Asthma and Allergy Center, inhaled hexamethonium as part of a research study on asthma. Shortly afterward she became mortally ill and died when her parents disconnected her from life support. In Roche's case researchers did not properly warn her about the risks she faced as a subject and didn't follow required procedures.[61]

Officials at Hopkins conducted an internal investigation and concluded that the doctor who performed the tests on Roche was primarily and personally at fault. But the Office for Human Research Protection took a close look at the procedures governing all the clinical trials at Johns Hopkins and took the unprecedented step of suspending for months every one of the federally funded clinical trials at the hospital and university. With Roche's death coming a little more than a year after hearings into Gelsinger's death, the move sent the unmistakable message to all sponsors of clinical trials that the FDA and OHRP were serious about enforcing regulations. The Johns Hopkins Medical School received more federal money for clinical trials than any other medical school in the country: $330 million per year for twenty-four hundred trials that enrolled more than fifteen thousand subjects.[62] While officials at Hopkins were contrite about Roche's death, they were angry about the penalty imposed by the OHRP.

After the funding was cut, Edward Miller, M.D., the CEO of Johns Hopkins Medicine (the name for all of Hopkins' medical enterprises, including the medical school) appeared on *The News-Hour with Jim Lehrer*. On the program Miller called the shutdown "draconian" and said that one death in one hundred years of conducting clinical trials at Johns Hopkins was a "pretty good track record."[63]

After the nationally renowned Baltimore school resumed its federally funded clinical trials program, changes were made to improve the process employed in its trials. One year later the school went from having one IRB to having six; it tripled the space devoted to conducting trials; it increased full-time staff from eight to twenty; it hired an outside auditor to organize paperwork; and it started educational classes for staff on consent procedures and clinical trials in general.[64] It also settled a lawsuit for an undisclosed amount with Ellen Roche's family and did not admit any wrongdoing.[65]

Although botched experiments receive the most media attention, clinical trials have a statistically low incidence of injury. Most often, the system works.

An independent board that examined Jesse Gelsinger's death concluded that while mistakes did happen in Gelsinger's case, the board still had overall confidence in the need to conduct clinical trials. Their report said: "Clinical trials are essential if medicine is to progress and the health of each generation is to be better than the last."[66]

Some clinical trials are horrific to contemplate but nonetheless worthwhile to undertake. An experiment on starvation at the close of World War II provided valuable information on how U.S. forces could provide food to mass numbers of people who were struggling to find provisions to survive in the rubble of war-torn Europe in 1945.

Ancel Keys, Ph.D., who invented K-rations to efficiently provide nutrition to combat forces, recruited thirty-six conscientious objectors in 1944 for the yearlong trial. The men were informed and aware of the difficulty of the undertaking. Keys severely restricted the men's diets for six months to replicate the conditions faced by people living in Europe at the time. He studied the physical, emotional, and psychological consequences of the imposed famine and then set about rehabilitating the men back to health in six months. The study was instrumental in K-rations successfully sustaining vast populations as Europe was rebuilt after the war. The landmark two-volume *Biology of Human Starvation* remains the definitive treatise on the subject and continues to provide useful insights into anorexia and the relationship between diet and overall health. Dr. Keys and the men who volunteered for the study have been hailed as selfless heroes for their work and sacrifice.[67]

Regulations are tough, but not because federal departments are heartless. There is flexibility built into the regulatory system so lives can be saved quickly. The FDA has an institutionalized, accelerated approval program to rush treatment to patients if a drug is particularly promising. In 2001 the agency released a leukemia drug in just three months.[68] In 2007, to help save the life of four-year-old cancer patient Penelope London, Speaker of the House

Nancy Pelosi and several legislators joined the FDA in advocating for the release of another promising but risky new drug. The FDA said it would not hold Neotropix, Inc., the small biotech company that makes the drug, liable if Penelope died. According to an article in the May 1, 2007, *Wall Street Journal*, even with the blessing of the FDA Neotropix refused to administer the drug to Penelope because of potential liability exposure.

Although government regulations are entrenched as an accepted part of clinical trials, there are still serious issues to address. Most of them are ethical considerations such as conflict of interest concerns about researchers who hold stock in pharmaceutical companies, incentives paid by drug companies to doctors to recruit subjects, manipulation of trial data, and informed consent by patients. These issues are more subtle than the dramatic abuses of the past and more difficult to regulate.

Some people have even questioned whether our system of patient protection actually protects patients. Doctors, for instance, have expressed deep reservations over the FDA's decision in 1998 to approve thalidomide for limited use to treat a severe and common dermatological condition caused by Hansen's disease (better known as leprosy). The drug, originally developed to treat morning sickness and other conditions, became notorious for causing severe birth defects in children in the early 1960s, most notably the development of infant "flipper arms." Thalidomide affected seventeen children born in the United States to mothers who took part in a 1959 clinical trial. As a result of the trial, the FDA blocked the drug from reaching U.S. pharmacy shelves. Even so, the drug was widely prescribed and available over the counter in Europe for many years.[69]

That history is why some doctors were alarmed in 1998 when the multinational pharmaceutical company Celgene reintroduced the drug in the United States after it was approved for off-label use to treat patients with conditions other than Hansen's disease. What would happen, doctors wondered, if a patient became pregnant while on thalidomide? Given thalidomide's past, some doctors insisted on unusually tight controls on the drug.

"Not all tragedies can be redeemed, but we can learn from all tragedies," warned George Annas, M.D., and Sherman Alias, M.D., in an article published in the *American Journal of Public Health* arguing for more intense government regulation of the drug. "The FDA has the responsibility to ensure that thalidomide is safely introduced in the United States. But physicians and patients must share responsibility for its proper use."[70]

There have also been concerns about whether the FDA allows pharmaceutical companies too much freedom in how they design trials and how they report the results of those trials. Pharmaceutical studies can be designed to falsely increase the likelihood of getting the results the drug company wants. "For example, they might use lower doses of a competitor's medication than might ordinarily be used in clinical practice, compared to the high dose of their medication," said Dr. Paul Appelbaum. "So, they get more of an effect with their medication, which they can then say is a success. These distortions creep in."[71]

Alleged attempts to manipulate clinical trial data led to the fiasco involving Vioxx, a painkiller from the pharmaceutical company Merck. In November 1998 Merck published the results of eight clinical trials on fifty-four hundred patients that showed the drug was safe. Based on that trial, the company asked the FDA to approve the drug. Before the FDA acted, however, Merck started another study on eight thousand people. It was called the Vioxx Gastrointestinal Outcomes Research study, or VIGOR. The trial was designed to determine if, among other things, the painkiller was gentler on the digestive system than naproxen. Vioxx's gentleness was potentially a main selling point of the new medication.[72]

In May 1999 the FDA approved Vioxx. Ten months later Merck published the results of the VIGOR study. They did not, however, publish the complete results. What they released showed that a small number of people taking the drug had suffered heart attacks during the trial; Merck reported the number of heart attacks at seventeen when it was actually twenty. They allegedly further tweaked the results by withholding other information about the cardiovascular impact of the drug.[73]

Cardiologists eventually took a hard look at the unabridged data from VIGOR and published a report that cast doubt on Vioxx's safety for patients with heart conditions. Additional studies reinforced their concern. In September 2004, after another study by Merck, the company took Vioxx off the market. They also opened the floodgates to years of lawsuits and potential corporate ruin. Later research estimated—but has not yet conclusively proven—that eighty-eight thousand Americans suffered heart attacks while on Vioxx and thirty-eight thousand of them died.[74]

The Vioxx story reveals how ethics have become more flexible and prone to interpretation when it comes to corporate involvement in the development of expensive drugs. But Merck isn't the only one that comes under criticism for Vioxx. The story also highlights the holes and limits in how well clinical trials are supervised. "I believe that there should be a full congressional review of this case," Eric J. Topol, M.D., of the Cleveland Clinic Foundation, wrote in a blistering opinion piece in the *New England Journal of Medicine* in 2004. "The senior executives at Merck and the leadership at the FDA share responsibility for not having taken appropriate action and not recognizing that they are accountable for the public health."[75] Litigation to decide blame, and possibly punishment, for researchers and executives at Merck over Vioxx continues to move through the courts in several states. Merck maintains that it did nothing improper.

Corporate interests are not the only factors at play, Topol said.

"Despite the best efforts of many investigators to conduct and publish meaningful independent research concerning the cardio-vascular toxicity of rofecoxib (as Vioxx is called), only the FDA is given the authority to act. In my view, the FDA's passive position of waiting for data to accrue is not acceptable, given the strong signals that there was a problem and the vast number of patients who were being exposed."[76]

(An interesting side note to Topol's article provides a glimpse of just how rough and downright confusing things can get when a doctor criticizes a drug company and a government agency that approves drugs. Less than three months after Topol's article was published *Fortune* magazine reported that Topol had an alleged conflict of interest that may have prompted him to call Merck and the FDA to task. He allegedly had ties to a hedge fund that had shorted Merck stock, betting it would plunge in value after the Vioxx fiasco. Topol denied any conflict. Whatever the merits of the story, the *Fortune* piece showed keen insight about clinical trials in general when it said Topol's alleged involvement with the hedge fund "illustrate[s] the conflicts that can emerge when doctors step outside the world of medicine and become entangled with Wall Street."[77])

There are many reasons internal vigilance is jeopardized during clinical trials. Vera Sharav, founder of the Alliance for Human Research Protection, a public interest watchdog group tracking biomedical issues, says that research today is too tied up with corporate interests and that companies fund too much research at hospitals, universities, and in private labs. Increased regulation gets compromised because the FDA is overwhelmed with all the data that flows from so many drug-company-sponsored trials.[78]

Ken Faulkner disagrees, believing that having 20 million people in trials produces more accurate data. "You need large numbers," Faulkner says. "The results are better with bigger numbers, as opposed to something that just shows up as a statistical anomaly because you only had a handful of people. With any sample, the larger the sample the more trustworthy the results."[79]

The vast amount of corporate investment in clinical trials within the last twenty years raises new and challenging ethical concerns. When a doctor receives $8,000 from a large medical company for recruiting a patient into a clinical trial, the level of patient care a doctor is providing could be compromised. Such incentives might affect how persuasively a doctor recruits patients and whether the best regard for the patient's health is being considered in light of a business deal that could enrich the doctor.[80]

Therapeutic misconception is also a significant issue and is thoroughly built in to how trials function today. It's not as simple and reductive as researchers twisting arms and misleading subjects in clinical trials. Subjects often mislead themselves. Some clinical trials candidates suffering from cancer, diabetes, asthma, and other life-threatening conditions sincerely believe that trials are a valid medical treatment option. "Subjects often come into clinical research studies believing that their own interests will be met in the same way as if they were receiving ordinary [medical] treatment," Appelbaum says. "They are really unaware of the differences between being in a study and receiving ordinary treatment. And there are lots of them. I think people are out there looking for a treatment that gives them some greater chance of symptom relief or cure depending on what their condition is. They've come to see clinical trials as a way of achieving that, particularly if they have not had success with more traditional forms of treatment."[81]

Although therapeutic misconception is accepted by most bioethicists and researchers as being widespread in clinical research, some believe medical care is actually provided more often than not in clinical trials. Ezekiel J. Emanuel, M.D., chair of the department of bioethics at the Clinical Center of the National Institutes of Health, says, "Therapeutic misconception is a very confused, elastic, over-generalized term. In a randomized, controlled trial I think it's very difficult for a patient to have a therapeutic misconception. If it's a . . . trial where one arm is standard care and one is research, it's very difficult for someone to say there's not going to be some benefit."[82]

Regardless, clinical trials are not designed to provide patients with quality care. Somehow, patient care became part of a process designed to only gather information. The doctor administering the trial might be wearing a stethoscope and a lab coat, but she's not there to cure anyone. She's there to collect information from a subject and learn more about medicine.

It's hard to rationally expect better than standard medical treatment during the course of a clinical trial when some trials don't succeed in providing improved care. Sometimes the medical community ends up more confused about treatment than they were before the clinical trial. In December 2005 the results of a clinical trial were released that studied whether tight control to keep blood sugar levels low in diabetics actually prevented heart attacks and strokes, as had long been supposed but had never been clinically proven. The seventeen-year-long, federally funded clinical trial tested more than fourteen hundred type I diabetic subjects aged thirteen to thirty-nine. Half the subjects went through intense therapy to keep their blood sugar rigorously controlled and the other half were less tightly controlled.[83]

Before the trial was finished researchers said they had some positive results. "It was amazing," said David Nathan, M.D., the cochairman of the study about the group that had well-controlled blood sugars. "Therapy for six and one-half years seems to have had a dramatic [positive] effect."[84]

By the end of the study the verdict was published in the *New England Journal of Medicine*: Conscientious blood sugar control prevented heart attacks and strokes in diabetics. Doctors altered their treatments to make sure that their diabetic patients were keeping their blood sugar levels as tightly controlled as possible over the long term. They started relying heavily on a blood test that measures sugar levels over a three-month period, called an A1c test, to gauge the control of both type 1 and type 2 diabetics. Insurance companies even paid doctors extra if they got their patients' blood sugar low.[85] Doctors said the results of the clinical trial would encourage wider use of existing tools, such as the A1c, and the development of new tools and therapies that would make a difference in people's lives.[86]

Two years and two months later, that study got turned on its head when another clinical trial was partially halted after results showed that diabetics who rigorously controlled and lowered their blood sugars *increased* their risk of death. Out of ten thousand type 2 diabetics middle-aged and older and enrolled in the federally funded study, there were fifty-four more deaths by heart attack in the group that tightly controlled their blood sugar than in the group that controlled their blood sugar less religiously.[87]

"It's confusing and disturbing that this has happened," said James Dove, M.D., president of the American College of Cardiology. "For fifty years, we've talked about getting blood sugar very low. Everything in the literature would suggest this is the right thing to do."[88] Other doctors said they were stunned by the results and in a quandary about how to treat their diabetic patients in the future.

Worse still, researchers didn't know what caused the results. The best conclusion that could be reached, although vague and noncommittal, was "clearly, people without diabetes are different from people who have diabetes and get their blood sugar low."[89]

Studies such as these show that, while not impossible, the odds are stacked against someone receiving better treatment through a trial. My chance, for instance, of being cured of diabetes in my clinical trial is probably in the same ballpark as my chance of winning $10,000 in the Powerball drawing: 1 in 584,431.[90] But, instead of a dollar, I have to put my life up as the bet.

The history of clinical trials shows great swings between significantly helping and dramatically harming people. The Vioxx experience highlights two hard and simple truths about clinical trials: They are the only way to discover for sure how a drug or treatment will work on people, and they involve great risk. The information doctors gather from testing on rodents/nonrodents, plotting charts in a lab, crunching numbers on a computer, creating statistical models, and graphing probabilities is not always applicable to people. In such a charged and constantly changing atmosphere, it's little wonder that ethics are not hard and fast in dictating what exactly is right and wrong in clinical trials.

"Legitimate researchers know that very few diseases, like cancer, are going to be conquered by the miracle discovery in the laboratory," Faulkner says. "It's the clinical trial year after year, where you slowly whittle away, that does it. Some forms of childhood leukemia had a 90 percent death rate and now, twenty-five years later, have an 80 percent cure rate. That's the result of years and years of whittling and whittling in lots of clinical trials, with a lot of people, and gradually improving. It's a lot of tweaking along the way. Although [breakthroughs] happen, it's usually not a revolutionary discovery. It's slogging it out in clinical trials."[91]

Today's regulations by the FDA and other agencies are a direct result of lessons learned in past trials. One expert, Howard Markel, M.D., Ph.D., of the Center for the History of Medicine at the University of Michigan, says the FDA was founded as a reaction to companies putting profits before health. And while it may seem like the same grab for profits with no regard for health is happening again, the system, although imperfect, is doing the dauntingly complicated job of keeping Americans protected while at the same time allowing medical innovation to move forward.

Modern governmental rules are the reason a clinical trial today usually doesn't involve doctors misleading patients for years or withholding lifesaving treatment, as with Tuskegee. Clinical trials are typically controlled experiments with expert care and supervision. But subjects still have to sign a disclaimer saying they understand they could die. In a time when people in the United States are more in charge of their own health care than ever before in human history and thoroughly vetted information is available at the click of a mouse, subjects should completely understand and appreciate that reality before they sign. That's because, despite the best regulations in the world, no government can control every aspect of an enterprise as risky as clinical trials. It always has been and always will be a crapshoot.

Chapter 3

MONEY MAKES THE TRIAL
GO 'ROUND

A FTER GIVING A PRESENTATION at the annual meeting of the American Society for Bioethics and Humanities
in Washington, D.C., David Satin, M.D., a renowned physician and
bioethicist from the University of Minnesota, points out an interesting thing about medicine and money. Look carefully, he says,
and notice that the farther away one gets from patients, the more
money one makes. "Nurses spend the most time with patients and
they make the least money. Doctors spend five, ten minutes with a
patient and they make more. Hospital CEOs and hospital administrators make more than doctors and they don't even see patients.
An insurance company makes more—they have contact with patients over the phone, but they're not in the same building as
them. The drug companies make the most money and they have
no contact with patients at all."[1]

Companies that actually conduct clinical trials are high in the
financial/medical pecking order. They have no contact with "patients" during clinical trials. They work with people as "subjects"
in order to generate data that is then used to get licensure to sell
medical products and drugs. The distinction is important because
clinical trials are usually more about money than medical discovery and patient care. And there's a lot of money in clinical trials.
As previously noted, they are a $24-billion-a-year industry in the
United States.[2] Even though it's enormous and growing, the

overall industry is not well understood by the government, the public, or even by those who conduct clinical trials. The standard business practices of clinical trials, if there are any, do not appear to be written down and agreed to by those involved in trials. Information and reporting about the industry is scattered and inconsistent. Individual aspects of the industry have been written about in medical journals, financial reports, and newspapers, but it has previously escaped close, comprehensive scrutiny. How exactly do clinical trials generate profits for companies? What kind of companies and which companies in particular make the profits? How much profit is made? The industry is so new that clear answers to those questions are hard to come by.

Most of the $24 billion a year goes to corporations, small companies, researchers, doctors, and other experts who conduct trials.[3] But advertising agencies, lawyers, colleges and universities, huge multinational conglomerates, private research companies, hospitals, doctors, and investigators profit from clinical trials as well.

Colleges, universities, and medical schools receive a relatively small portion of the money—certainly much smaller than they used to get—because most clinical trials no longer take place in hospitals or research institutions. In the last twenty-five years, as the pharmaceutical industry has grown, clinical trials started moving from the halls of academe to the cubicles of private companies.[4] Almost 75 percent of all the money spent on designing and conducting clinical trials in the United States is spent by corporations.[5] Much of that money is invested in clinical trials by pharmaceutical companies that have championed privatizing clinical trials, which has given pharmaceutical companies more control over how studies are carried out. The shift toward privatized trials in the last two decades was made because for-profit companies completed trials faster and cheaper than academic medical institutions.[6] That's crucial for pharmaceutical companies because in the drug development business time equals a staggering amount of money. The moment any new drug is patented—before clinical trials start—a twenty-year clock starts ticking toward when the patent expires.[7] When the patent ends, the drug company's monopoly on the drug ends and the medication can be sold by anyone as a generic. Each day that a drug is being tested in a clinical trial is a day taken away from the window of time it can be sold exclusively to consumers. And just one of those days can cost a pharmaceutical company millions. In 2003, for instance, the top-selling prescription medication in the world was Pfizer's cholesterol-lowering drug, Lipitor, with sales of $9.2 billion.[8] That's more than $25 million in sales *every single day*.

But before Pfizer sold the very first tablet of Lipitor to some guy diagnosed with elevated HDL, they first had to find subjects for clinical trials that were needed to test the drug and prove to the FDA it was safe and effective. Finding subjects who are specifically qualified for a particular clinical trial is a time-consuming, frustrating, and expensive effort.

The drug company sponsoring the clinical trial will often hire a clinical research organization, or CRO, to do the actual work of recruiting subjects and carrying out the clinical trial. If they're testing a new diabetes drug, for example, the CRO starts off by purchasing the names and addresses of ten thousand diabetics, usually from data-gathering companies that build such lists from a variety of sources such as magazine subscriptions, survey responses, even the club card consumers use at pharmacies and supermarkets. So many names are purchased because the CROs have to cast as wide a net as possible when trawling for potential subjects. They're not only looking for diabetics who meet specific symptomatic criteria to fit the study, they're also working against a very small response rate to such inquiries. A letter is then mailed to those ten thousand people, asking the potential subjects if they want to take part in the study. Usually the response rate is 2 percent. That means two hundred people will call to say they're interested in being in the study. Out of those, one hundred will be disqualified after a phone interview when they don't fit the criteria for the trial because they're overweight, their diabetes is too severe, they drink too much, or have some other issue that culls them from consideration. The one hundred people remaining are invited to come in to the CRO office for an exam. Only half will show up so now it's down to fifty people. Out of those fifty, the physical exam will eliminate half of those as unsuitable. At the end of the process, only twenty-five out of ten thousand people will end up in the trial as subjects.[9] Once the study begins, things get worse. One out of four subjects in clinical trials drops out before the trial ends.[10]

This anemic conversion rate poses a real challenge for companies and institutions conducting clinical trials because, for a variety of reasons, they need more subjects than ever before. To avoid the after-market problems that arose with Vioxx and other drugs, the FDA is now requiring that a greater number of subjects be enrolled in every clinical trial to gain a more accurate picture of the drug's potential side effects before it's sold. More trials are also being launched because drug companies have been taking one drug and applying it to treat multiple conditions. Each of those new applications requires a new round of clinical trials. When the antidepressant drug Wellbutrin, for example, was discovered to also curb nicotine cravings, it was altered slightly and marketed as a prescription drug to help people stop smoking. That "new" drug, Zyban, then had to be tested in new clinical trials.

Further adding to the need for more subjects is that more drugs are being developed than ever before. There is an estimated 52 percent increase in the number of new drugs entering clinical trials since 2000.[11] Aging baby boomers are requiring more meds; chronic conditions, such as asthma and diabetes, have increased significantly in the past decade; thanks to improved technology, doctors are diagnosing and treating those chronic diseases with medications more often than they did in the past; even the new

Medicare Part D drug-coverage plan contributes to the increase. People are also simply buying more drugs. The Kaiser Family Foundation reports that between 1994 and 2005 the average number of prescriptions per person in the United States increased from 7.9 to 12.3.[12]

To sell all these new drugs, starting in the early 1990s pharmaceutical companies significantly stepped up their direct-to-consumer advertising. They ramped up how much they spend to advertise drugs from $1.1 billion in 1997 to $4.2 billion in 2005.[13] While the billions invested in television, radio, newspaper, and magazine ads is helping drive demand, that isn't the only reason for so many new drugs. In the past twenty-five years the United States has become a consumer culture when it comes to medicine: People are not only buying more drugs and looking for new treatments, they are demanding them. If doctors won't prescribe the new drugs and treatments they want, some will change doctors or use other means to get them on their own.

Sam Hutchinson, for instance, takes forty-four pills a day and only a few of them are prescribed by his doctor.[14] Medications are chosen for the seven-year-old cancer patient by his father, Neil Hutchinson, a defense-contractor recruiter, whose medical background consists mostly of finding new drugs on the Internet so he can create a drug "cocktail" to treat his son's cancer. Some of the medicine in the anticancer cocktail that Sam gets each day is either still in the animal-testing phase, meant for other illnesses, or has not gone through clinical trials at all. Neil explains that he needs to play "lab rat" with his son because without the kind of self-directed intervention he is undertaking his son would most likely die.[15]

Hutchinson is not a member of some self-prescribing fringe element. He's part of a small but growing trend of patients and their families who go on the Internet, find out about new drugs and treatments as they are first coming to light, and do whatever they can to get hold of those drugs and treatments to try and save their own life or the life of a loved one. The few doctors who are in favor of self-treatment for cancer say they are approached by up to a dozen patients a week who want to go that route rather than receive traditional doctor-prescribed care.[16]

Self-treatment is not limited to cancer. A Web site called PatientsLikeMe.com has thousands of members who share information about what medications and treatments they are receiving. Special software on the site then converts that information into charts and graphs to display the effects of what patients are doing. Other patients study the data so they can either change their own courses of treatment or actively collaborate with their doctors to alter their care. "The 7,000 members of PatientsLikeMe, in other words, are beta testers—they may be the vanguard of how we all will care and treat our résumé of chronic diseases," according to the *New York Times* in a story about the site. "They're not typical patients, in the sense of waiting for advice from a doctor. They are, rather, copractitioners treating their conditions and guiding their care, with possibly profound implications."[17]

The practice of creating cancer treatment cocktails and having patients treat themselves takes place despite warnings that real damage, up to and including death, can result from taking untested drugs or untested combinations of drugs. Hutchinson tries to mitigate the possibility of disaster for his son by taking the medications Sam receives himself to gauge their effects.[18]

People running clinical trials would rather see self-treating subjects, like the Hutchinsons, enrolled in trials.[19] Whether this trend indicates a decline in the numbers of people enrolling in clinical trials remains to be seen. What it already indicates is that there is an intense and growing demand, especially from those who are sick with chronic conditions like diabetes, arthritis, heart disease and others, for new drugs and therapies.

There even have been situations where people have taken

pharmaceutical companies to court demanding to be treated with experimental drugs. In 2003 thirty-four subjects in a clinical trial to treat Parkinson's disease underwent surgery as part of a clinical trial. Two holes were drilled in subjects' heads and two pumps were implanted into their stomachs with catheters going to the brain delivering an experimental drug to treat their Parkinson's. For some, the drug worked wonders. Then, in 2004, the drug company Amgen shut down the trial, saying the drug might be ineffective and even harmful. Subjects in the trial sued Amgen so they could keep receiving the experimental drug.

Roger Perlmutter, M.D., the executive vice president of research and development at Amgen, says that subjects who received a placebo appeared to do as well as patients who received the drug. Also, studies on monkeys showed they had lesions on the parts of the brain that control movement and balance after taking the drug. Given those developments, Perlmutter says he didn't think it was ethical to keep giving the subjects the drug.[20] The subjects say it wasn't ethical for Amgen to stop giving them the drug. They filed a lawsuit to get the drug back because they claimed it was effective in controlling their Parkinson's symptoms. Many of the subjects enrolled in the study said the "treatment" diminished the spasms and shaking common in Parkinson's, that they were able to walk normally, stand straight up, talk more clearly, even be intimate with their spouses. One man said after being on the drug that for the first time in years he could smell his wife's home cooking.[21]

Patient advocacy groups also took up the cause and rallied to demand that the trial be restarted. "We think there is kind of a moral pact that one makes with a company in these situations that gives the patients a privilege of having continued access to treatment," Robin Anthony Elliott, executive director of the Parkinson's Disease Foundation, said.[22]

Courts are still wrestling with whether the subjects will get "treatment" again from Amgen and whether the company is under any moral, ethical, or legal obligation to "treat" the subjects. One health-care ethicist says the Amgen case presents an area of research that is not "settled" but is being raised more and more. If courts or government agencies decide that sponsors of clinical trials are obliged to provide treatment after a clinical trial is completed, then drug development might be significantly reduced.[23]

Until those decisions are made, the number of new drugs and medical technologies will only keep increasing as biotech companies delve into the human genome, stem-cell therapies, and medical applications for DNA. In 2007 alone there were four hundred products developed by biotech firms that are in late-stage clinical trials testing[24] and there are many more on the way.

One thing, however, that might keep these potentially fantastic discoveries from being sold to consumers in little brown plastic bottles is the lack of suitable subjects to test them. Even though more people than ever before are enrolling in clinical trials as subjects, demand is outstripping supply. That's why recruitment has become a major part of the clinical trials industry and why people increasingly see and hear actual TV ads like this one:

> Do you suffer from chronic low back pain? Are you currently taking pain medication for your lower back pain? If so, you may qualify for a research study of an investigational medication for chronic low back pain. Participants must be between the ages of 21 and 75 and suffer from chronic low back pain. If qualified, you will receive all study-related care and investigational medication at no cost and be compensated for time and travel. Call now for more information and to see if you qualify.[25]

This ad is a fairly typical thirty-second television commercial recruiting subjects to test an experimental drug in a clinical trial.

In the spot, words appear on the screen to mirror the text as it is narrated. A photo of a woman in her forties remains onscreen throughout the ad. She has a hand on her lower back and she's wincing in discomfort. It's an image anyone who has ever had back problems can immediately identify and sympathize with. It communicates to the lower back pain sufferer that whoever sponsored this ad really understands what people with lower back pain endure. By inference it says that whoever sponsored this ad is dedicated to finding a successful medical treatment for the millions who endure this debilitating condition.

At first glance the words in the ad seem like unremarkable boilerplate, like an innocuous, familiar pitch, until you start to really examine them. The language suggests that the lower back pain sufferer who signs up for the study might "qualify" for something, like they might win some sort of prize. The "participant" might be "compensated." It says the subjects can even "receive all study-related care and investigational medication at no cost."

The words "clinical trial," "subject," test," and "experimental" never appear in the ad. The potential subject is called a "participant." The clinical trial is called a "research study." The words are carefully chosen.

In all advertising, exact wording is crucial in trying to motivate a person to take the action desired by the company placing the ad. Using specific images and words to motivate action is the very purpose of advertising. It's the same whether McDonald's is trying to convince you to buy a Big Mac or a company is trying to convince you to volunteer for a clinical trial. And in the clinical trials industry, the vocabulary that might convince a person to enroll in a study is very well studied.

In a 1994 review of clinical trials consent forms (the paperwork a person signs, after being informed of the risks, in which they agree to the terms of the trial and to enroll in the trial) presented to nineteen hundred potential subjects "direct evidence of language used to deceive potential research subjects" was found.[26] In that same independent review by a panel studying radiation experiments conducted by the U.S. government from 1944 to 1974, the subjects who made the decision to take part in the studies were interviewed and surveyed about what convinced them to enroll. They told interviewers what they thought of terms used instead of "research study," including "clinical trial," "clinical investigation," "medical study," and "medical experiment." Subjects thought "medical experiment" was the most negative term. They found the term "medical research" only a little better than "clinical investigation" and "clinical trial." The term that most strongly motivated patients to enroll in the study was "medical research," which is a close cousin to the words "research study" used in the recruitment ad for the lower back pain clinical trial.[27]

The reason that "medical research" was the big winner was because, compared to the other phrasing, patients view a research study as "less risky, as less likely to involve unproven treatments, and as offering a greater chance at medical benefits."[28] In other words, people think by enrolling in medical research they have a better chance of receiving treatment for an ailment rather than just being a research subject. That inference is the "therapeutic misconception" in action.

One theory as to why such careful wording is used in consent forms might also explain why the words are so carefully chosen in ads recruiting subjects for clinical trials. As bioethicist Dr. George Annas puts it, "Medicine . . . is currently faced with a new dominant ideology—the ideology of the marketplace, which puts profit making . . . as its highest priority."[29]

Annas points out that the pharmaceutical industry has seen the largest, steadiest annual growth of any industry since the 1940s. The emerging biotechnology industry, which is pushing the need for even more clinical trials, is also heating up the competition in the drug business.[30] That means clinical trials loom as a bottleneck that can strangle profitability if subjects are not moved through them quickly and efficiently. In such an atmosphere, using specific words that have already been judged more, rather than less, likely to get subjects through the door to a clinical trial is a powerful contributor to the bottom line. It is, after all, called "patient recruitment" not "subject recruitment."

The FDA has been rigorously monitoring and regulating direct-to-consumer advertising by drug companies on television and radio, and in magazines and newspapers, since 1962.[31] In early 1997 Congress held hearings in which the regulations for advertising prescription drugs to consumers were debated.[32] There are, however, no standard guidelines making sure the advertising to recruit subjects is not misleading.

Criticism of their medical ads forced Pfizer to pull a popular, two-year-long television campaign in 2008. The advertising featured the pioneer in the development of the artificial heart, Robert Jarvik, M.D., touting Lipitor, Pfizer's cholesterol-lowering medication that was believed to help prevent heart attacks. It seemed like an advertising match made in medical heaven. Pfizer paid Jarvik $1.35 million to be filmed while he was rowing a catamaran on a river and otherwise looking fit and trim as he explained how Lipitor was good for your heart. Several details in the spot were questionable—the rower was a body double. Also, Jarvik, who is a doctor, is not a cardiologist, and he was described as the "inventor of the artificial heart" although scientists who worked on the heart with Jarvik said that credit shouldn't go to Jarvik alone. Members of a congressional committee studying medical advertising thought the ad was misleading. Before the criticism could reach a deafening roar or result in fines, Pfizer chose to cease the ad campaign.[33]

The television ad that recruited subjects for the back pain study never made it clear who was sponsoring the ad. Was a doctor, a researcher, or a pharmaceutical company soliciting people for the research study? The ad was created and produced not by a medical research organization, but by an advertising agency that specializes in recruiting patients for clinical trials. That's a good indicator of just how much money there is to be made in clinical trials.

Clinical Trial Media, an ad agency that specializes in subject recruitment, created the back pain television spot. The company describes itself as "The media-buying specialists for patient recruitment advertising."[34] They have a staff of twenty-two people in their Jericho, New York, office. The company has estimated sales of $1.6 million per year.[35] They also have competition. A few of the many other agencies that specialize in subject recruitment advertising are Axiom Marketing, Inc., Trial Builder, BBK Patient Recruitment, and MMG, whose slogan is "We Get Patients."[36] These aren't just small mom-and-pop companies. MMG, along with another agency called Corbett Accel Healthcare Group, is owned by Diversified Agency Services. DAS, in turn, is owned by Omnicom Group.[37] At the end of 2006 Omnicom was the number one media conglomerate in the world with sixty-six thousand employees worldwide, more than $11 billion in revenue, and an annual revenue growth rate of 8.5 percent.[38] Omnicom became such a corporate behemoth by buying and investing in companies like MMG, that serve expanding sectors of the economy.

Even though these ad agencies specialize in recruiting people to test new drugs, medical devices, and procedures, they describe themselves more in financial terms than in scientific terms. In the patient recruitment business, topics like subject satisfaction; the success rate of the new drug, device, or procedure; science; and health care take a backseat to concerns about money.

The top management for Clinical Trial Media, for instance, is composed of former advertising executives. According to their company overview, CTM has more than ten years of experience in subject recruitment advertising, has spent $400 million on recruitment advertising, and has successfully enrolled fifteen hundred trials for their clients. In a trial to study osteoarthritis of the knee and hip that required enrolling subjects at thirty-eight sites, CTM launched a TV campaign and generated 3,962 calls from interested potential subjects. In four weeks the campaign enrolled eighty-one patients and helped the client meet their recruitment goal. The cost of meeting that goal was $4,275 per subject,[39] or $346,274 all told.

But who exactly is spending all this money to get subjects?

National Clinical Research is in a ten thousand-square-foot facility in an office park off Interstate 64 in Richmond, Virginia. Patients sign in at NCR, as it's better known, and take a seat in a waiting room lit by table lamps. While they wait for their name to be called they leaf through copies of *People* magazine, listen to a soft rock radio station, watch TV, or admire the impressionist-style prints on the walls. Once called, they're escorted by a nurse into one of the fourteen exam rooms and are seen by one of the specialists on the thirty-person staff, including a full-time dietician or one of the two doctors who are on the premises at all times. Depending on what they're there for, patients during their exam have access to scales that are accurate to a tenth of a pound, a machine that measures bone density to the exact millimeter, even a $250,000 Accutron that takes an image of blood vessels with sound waves to measure lining density and plaque buildup.

More than three thousand people a year come through NCR's doors, about the same number in a typical doctor's practice.[40] NCR, however, is not a doctor's practice. It's a CRO, one of thousands of private companies in the United States that conducts and manages clinical trials research for money. CROs are such a new business sector that their trade association is only five years old. There doesn't even seem to be an agreed-upon name for what the acronym CRO stands for: "clinical research organization," or "contract research organization" as they are also called because they are typically subcontractors for large pharmaceutical companies.

CROs conduct 77 percent of all clinical trials carried out in the world. The industry boasts estimated sales of $10 billion per year,[41] close to half of all the money generated in the clinical trials industry. With an annual growth rate between 14 and 16 percent per year, those numbers are going up.[42] Whether CROs are a positive influence in health care is the subject of intense debate between CROs and researchers in academe, who are skeptical of whether CROs benefit anything other than the bottom line of multinational corporations.

Further muddling the issue is the existence of smaller companies—such as National Clinical Research—that subcontract for CROs. These companies carry out much of the actual work, like patient recruitment, blood testing, etcetera, required of a clinical trial. The results of that work are sent to CROs that interpret the data and present the results to the sponsors of a clinical trial. Such smaller companies are CRO "sites," but they're frequently referred to as, or call themselves, CROs. That makes it hard to even know how many CROs and CRO sites there are doing business.

"I'm going to say—it's an increasing number—but I would think there are probably on the order of twenty or so full-service, global CROs," says Doug Peddicord, the director of the industry's trade group, the Association of Clinical Research Organizations (ACRO). "They provide Phase I through Phase IV services. Now, there is a much larger number of smaller companies that maybe are not global, or do not provide that full range of services etcetera, and that call themselves CROs.

"They are really not sites. I think I've seen numbers, in terms of the number of companies that describe themselves as CROs, as on the order of 600 to 800 in the U.S. and on the order of 1,000 to 1,500 worldwide. The numbers are very soft."

Whatever you call them and however many there are, CROs are a dynamic and controversial force in health care.

NCR is one of more than a thousand CRO "sites" in the United States that contract with CRO to conduct private clinical trials. The CRO industry was born in the mid-1980s when drug companies figured out they could get trials completed faster than at universities and research hospitals. To speed the process, drug companies turned to private companies that would do the trials. That meant everything including, but not limited to, recruiting subjects, hiring staff to conduct the trials, overseeing medical testing, gathering data from the trials, reporting the data to the FDA, and much more.

The people who set up CROs and CRO sites in the 1980s tended to come from either the world of academe or pharmaceutical research. From whichever setting, both sets of these business innovators shared a common realization. They saw that a new business model that delivers increased efficiency and speed in testing drugs was needed because academic medical institutions were not getting the job done fast enough.[43]

James McKenney, a Virginia native and a doctor of pharmacology, comes from the academic side of the CRO tracks. He left the Medical College of Virginia and started National Clinical Research in the early 1980s. At NCR he could conduct the kind of research he was already doing for the college but on his own terms, for a profit, and without the academic bureaucracy. He also started NCR because the kind of research he liked doing isn't a priority at academic medical institutions. He says such places are not designed or equipped to efficiently conduct routine drug trials. They are very good at discovery research, the kind of tinkering that brings about breakthroughs in medical science.

"Testing a new cholesterol drug is really cool to me," he says. "I like the idea that we can advance science, that we can advance the products that are available to people that make a difference in their lives, a fundamental difference in their lives in survival and quality of life. This is not chicken liver. It's good stuff. But it's routine, it's methodical, it's crank-and-turn. At a university that's not a rewarded input. You're rewarded if you're discovering new knowledge and advancing knowledge rather than participating in the advancement of a pharmaceutical company product."[44]

When you ask McKenney who pays his company for what it does, he answers very simply, "The drug company."[45]

The "crank-and-turn" way in which CRO sites make money is a pretty straightforward business deal between the drug company and the site. A CRO will develop a trial protocol with the sponsor of the trial, usually a pharmaceutical company or a biotech firm. Then they'll call a site, like NCR, with the specific parameters and the design of the clinical trial. They may want thirty subjects enrolled with ten visits per subject each, with ten blood draws, ten physical exams, and five EKGs over the course of those visits. They may also ask for data collection or sorting. The people at the site will essentially take their order and run their calculations on how much it will cost them to conduct the trial and how much profit they can make from the trial. Included in their costs are recruitment advertising, perhaps paying a fee to physicians who deliver a subject for a trial (a practice that still goes on but is declining in recent years[46]), staff, overhead, insurance, and whatever else they have to spend to conduct the trial according to the protocol. The site will then call the CRO and give them a figure of how much it will cost, say three thousand dollars per patient. If that's agreed to then a deal is made; the site is contracted and starts recruiting subjects and conducting the trial. If a subject drops out before the end of the trial, the site may get only a portion of the three thousand dollars.[47] The CRO, meanwhile, makes its profit by charging the drug company or biotech firm, in comparison, $4,000 per patient. The drug company sponsoring the trial takes all the financial risk if the trial doesn't produce the desired results or if it turns out the drug is not marketable. That risk can be enormous.

In 2006 Pfizer pulled the plug on a clinical trial for a heart attack prevention drug called torcetrapib. The medication was invented by a Pfizer researcher in 1992. It promised to lower bad cholesterol and, when combined with Pfizer's drug Lipitor, raise so-called good cholesterol in patients. Subjects were first given torcetrapib in 1992 and large-scale clinical trials with fifteen thousand subjects started in 2000, one year after Pfizer started construction on a $90 million facility in Ireland to manufacture what looked to be a blockbuster drug. In 2004 Pfizer published the results of a trial on nineteen patients in the *New England Journal of Medicine* that showed the drug was effective at preventing heart attacks. Things looked positive for the drug and for Pfizer. Then in late 2005 the same clinical trial showed that the drug raised subjects' blood pressure. In 2005 the drug's development was stopped when eighty-two people who took it in a clinical trial died compared to fifty-one deaths among people in the trial who took a placebo. Pfizer's $1 billion investment to develop the drug was a complete loss.[48]

While the business end of things is fairly straightforward, the ethical, medical, and scientific implications of the clinical trials business are more controversial especially when trials are not stopped before something goes seriously wrong.

In 2006 the fifth largest global CRO, PAREXEL International, was running a trial to study an antibody when six of the eight previously healthy participants in a Phase I study being conducted in Great Britain landed in intensive care after suffering multiple organ failure.[49] British investigators didn't directly blame the U.S.-based PAREXEL for the sudden organ shutdowns, but investigators from Great Britain's Medicines and Healthcare products Regulatory

Agency appointed a group of experts to study whether tougher regulations were needed to safeguard subjects in similar trials.[50]

In October 2007 an article in the *New England Journal of Medicine* examined the risks and benefits of CROs dominating the clinical trials industry.[51] The story, which was critical of CROs, apparently touched some nerves and set off a spat between academic research institutions and commercial research institutions.

The article, by Miriam Shuchman, M.D., says "surprisingly little attention" has been paid to how CROs have taken over much of academe's function in conducting clinical trials.[52] She writes in the article about trials in which people were severely injured; where there were apparent conflicts of interest between pharmaceutical company executives and regulators in the FDA; where there was what some call the inadequate training of CRO employees; and in which ideas were put forth for better regulating how CROs functioned.[53] She quotes an economist as saying that the "commodification" of clinical trials "had begun to 'kill' clinical research."[54]

The Association for Clinical Research Organizations was not happy about the article. In a letter to the *Journal*'s editors, and also posted on ACRO's Web site, Executive Director Peddicord wrote, "CROs bring experience, efficiency and specialization to the drug development process. To assert that this specialized expertise has begun 'to kill' clinical research is unwarranted, and no empirical data is provided to support such a claim."[55]

An article in *ClinPage*, a business-to-business trade publication for the commercial clinical trials industry, took a much harder position than Peddicord. It said, "Part of the *NEJM*'s motivation for its article may be sour grapes in academia about the loss of billions of dollars in projects to CROs," because academic institutions just "can't get the job done for industry."[56]

Not efficiently enough getting "the job done for industry"

is the prevailing reputation academic research institutions have in the world of corporate pharmaceuticals. By contrast, CROs are thought by advocacy groups—such as Public Citizen—to be so deep in the pocket of big pharmaceutical companies that they routinely chase money at the expense of achieving verifiable, accurate scientific results.[57]

One way they could get the job done better and improve both of their images would be to become full partners in clinical research. Such relationships might benefit all parties. CROs and drug companies could pump massive amounts of money into academic institutions so they could pursue cutting-edge, and expensive, medical experimentation. The CROs and drug companies would be rewarded with access to the cachet and scientific knowledge of prestigious academic research institutions that they were criticized in the *New England Journal of Medicine* for sorely lacking.

That, however, isn't happening in any significant way. Instead academic institutions, feeling the economic pinch, are starting to look at how they can expand their role in commercial clinical trials. The feud between the *NEJM* and ACRO is just one indicator of how intense the head-to-head competition between academic institutions and CROs is becoming in the quest to snag lucrative corporate contracts. Academic research institutions may never get back to handling up to 80 percent of all clinical trials for corporations, but they are aggressively looking to haul in more than the 30 percent they get now.[58]

Academic institutions such as Duke University, the University of Rochester, and the University of Pittsburgh Medical Center Health System are starting CRO-academic hybrids to create a one-stop point of contact for drug companies, academic-based researchers, and community physicians who recruit patients and conduct some trials. Other medical schools are coming together and offering their services to big pharmaceutical companies as a consortium. Columbia University, Cornell University, and New

York Presbyterian Hospital put together the Clinical Trials Network. The director of the network, Michael Leahy, says, "Our goal is to take clinical research back from for-profit companies. We are trying to formulate a real alternative to the for-profit drug-trial entrepreneurs."[59]

Remarkably, there is no data and there have been no studies comparing the effectiveness and safety of clinical trials conducted at academic research institutions and those conducted by CROs. There are several possible explanations why such a study hasn't been done. That kind of comparative study would be expensive and difficult to undertake because in order to accurately compare results, the two trials would have to be conducted simultaneously and with the same exact protocols.[60] CROs are also loath to be open about their methods and results because they want to protect trade secrets. Academic research institutions competing with other universities and CROs also keep information close to the vest to maintain their competitive advantage.[61] And which side would pay for such a study? CROs would stand to lose even more credibility and academic institutions could lose their advantage over CROs, which is the commonly held belief that their methods are more stringent and their results more trustworthy than those of CROs.

Despite their tough talk, the two sides do join hands to achieve their common goals in some areas. In the islet cell transplant trial at the University of Virginia, for instance, subjects are supplied with expensive immunosuppression drugs direct from Wyeth Laboratories. The arrangement lets Wyeth test their drugs on islet transplant subjects, and the clinical trials team is able to supply a drug that is so expensive it would eliminate many qualified candidates from the study if they had to pay for it themselves.

While that's a win–win situation, another instance of how the two sides cooperate raises serious concerns about whether the influence of corporate money on clinical research is a positive one.

It used to be that principal investigators designed clinical trials before looking for a company to sponsor their research. These doctors and other experts, usually with medical backgrounds, laid out every aspect of the trial. Called a protocol, these plans include how many and what kind of people will be tested, a schedule of the testing procedures, including what kinds of drugs will be administered and in what doses, and how long the trial will last.[62] Other steps in the clinical trials process that may be included in the protocol are how the data from the trial will be collected and analyzed, how that information will be submitted to the FDA for review, and then how the results will be published in peer review journals so doctors, participants in the trial, and others can learn about the results. After designing the study the principal investigator would go looking for the money to make this expensive proposition happen. He or she would knock on drug companies' doors to see if they wanted to sponsor the trial. If the corporation signed on they would get a piece of the action should the drug get FDA approval and hit pharmacy shelves.

That model has been completely turned upside down. Today, in the new world of clinical trials, a study's design usually originates with corporations. Drug companies frequently design studies themselves then go looking for principal investigators to carry out the work. If the company doesn't have in-house experts to design a trial, the company will sometimes hire a principal investigator to design it based on the drug company's criteria.[63] There can even be several investigators for each study, one for each site where a trial is being conducted.[64]

This kind of cozy relationship building has succeeded in generating more accurate data from clinical trials sponsored by corporations than might be gathered if such experts were not on board. It's also stirred up a lot of conflict about the impact of corporate money on clinical trials.

The infusion of cash for clinical trials starting in the mid-1980s is what has caused this flip in the process. Whether the principal investigator is hired by the drug company to design a study or to carry out the company's design, that principal investigator is working for the drug company. Such arrangements raise questions about conflicts of interest; about whether the principal investigator is working in the interest of science and discovery or in the interest of their own pocketbook and the drug company filling it.

On the rare occasions when an investigator comes to a pharmaceutical company with a trial design, the company often sends it to their marketing department for their opinion on whether the company should take on the trial. Doctors' claims that clinically important drugs should be studied after FDA approval or after they are on pharmacy shelves (such as the postmarketing trials that uncovered problems with Vioxx) have been rejected by pharmaceutical companies because the results had the potential to cut into sales.[65]

Some authors and doctors claim that drug companies may skew the design of clinical trials so their drugs will come out looking more effective or less dangerous than they are. Among the tricks that can be used are testing the drug in a healthier population than will be taking the drug and comparing the new medication to a lower dose of an existing medication so the results look better for the drug being tested.[66]

Once the trial is finished—even when it's conducted openly and aboveboard—the focus shifts to how the data from the trial is analyzed and made public. This is one of the most crucial steps in the clinical trials process. The results are what matter most to the FDA when it is reviewing the drug for approval; to other researchers seeking to learn more about a particular medication and how it can be applied to treat people; to physicians who will be prescribing the drug; to the public who will be taking the drug and want to be aware of side effects and how well it works; and, of course, to the people who participated in the clinical trial.

Data from clinical trials conducted by companies and CROs is usually controlled by the company or the CRO rather than by the principal investigator. The principal investigator might not even get to see all the data. A physician-executive at one pharmaceutical company said the data was usually withheld because "some investigators want to take the data beyond where [it] should go."[67]

For academic researchers the results—or data—of a trial registered with the FDA traditionally are published in peer-reviewed journals, such as the *New England Journal of Medicine*, or in the National Library of Medicine database of clinical trials. This allows researchers and physicians open review of the trial so they can independently verify the results and methodology to judge for themselves if those results are sound and accurate. Publishing results, however, has become a tightly controlled proposition. That's because the results of a clinical trial don't *have* to be published. Because CROs and corporations own the data, trials conducted by them that yield negative results are not always published for review in a timely fashion if at all.

In the case of clinical trials for antidepressants conducted between 1987 and 2004, drug companies often didn't bother to publish the results from trials if they showed their drugs were not as effective as expected. An analysis released in 2008 of seventy-four clinical trials for twelve antidepressants revealed that 94 percent of the trials that yielded positive results for the drugs were published whereas only 14 percent of the unfavorable results were.[68]

Harlan Krumholz, M.D., of Yale University, took the extraordinary step of blowing the whistle on two drug companies he says were hiding something when they chose to withhold trial results for two years on the cholesterol-lowering drugs Vytorin and Zetia. The drugs were blockbuster sellers with more than 3 million prescriptions for each written each month and sales of more than $5 billion in 2007.[69] In April 2008 Krumholz released internal e-mail messages from Merck and Schering-Plough, the makers of the drugs, indicating they kept preliminary results of trials secret when the studies showed that neither of the drugs worked exactly the way in which the companies claimed they did. The companies explained the delay at the time by saying images of arteries taken to measure cholesterol buildup were unclear and more testing would need to be done. Krumholz said the trial results, when they were finally published, meant the drugs shouldn't be used for treatment except as "a last resort."[70] Two large cardiology associations agreed with Krumholz and made the same recommendation. When that news was released Merck shares fell 15 percent and Schering's lost 26 percent.[71]

Krumholz views the stock losses as nothing more than a correction to overpriced shares. While he is quick to say there are many good researchers and doctors doing valuable clinical trials research in corporate settings, he agrees that the influence of money in medicine brings in a new, outside influence that could cause some people and companies to be more concerned with the bottom line than with the science. Luckily, Krumholz says, it's fortunate in this era of big medical money that more and more people are keeping a closer eye on clinical trials results and methods: "I think the companies and others who conduct clinical trials are under greater scrutiny than ever before. Now, if a person notices something, they have the means to say something about it. Before they had to convince a reporter to write a story but now they can post information on a blog or on the Internet and people start taking a harder look at what's going on."[72]

So much attention has become focused on how trials are designed and then selectively published that leading peer-reviewed medical journals took a stand in 2007 to not publish articles about studies unless full results had been released on the National Medical Library's public database of results.

In 2007 that awareness also led to a trade group representing large pharmaceutical companies to, on their own, publish more results in a more timely fashion on their public database as well. However, full disclosure of all trials' results is not mandatory and companies continue to be under no obligation to release complete results from the trials they sponsor.[73] "There was legislation considered that once a trial is registered it should be published in two years," Krumholz says. "That's very generous. But, I don't think it went anywhere."[74]

When results are published as an article in a recognized medical journal, there's no telling who wrote the article. Some articles that bear the investigator's name are actually authored by a writer who isn't even involved in the trial. Instead, the writer is hired by the CRO or drug company, and he or she receives a packet of information and writes the article based on that information. A drug industry executive dismissed any sinister overtones about the practice by saying that ghostwriters are capable, professional, and well trained; that principal investigators are often too busy to write the articles themselves; and that if there are any errors in such articles it's the investigator's fault because he is responsible for carefully reviewing any article with his name on it before it goes out.[75] "Ghostwriting has been going on probably forever," Krumholz says. "Now, however, at least there's a growing awareness about the practice."[76]

Another area raising questions about how corporate money might be influencing clinical trials is the practice by some pharmaceutical companies of paying doctors for each patient they recruit into a company-sponsored trial. At one academic medical institution there was a 300 percent increase over fourteen years in the number of principal investigators who had financial ties to companies sponsoring their research.[77]

Corporate influence is so pervasive that esteemed academic medical institutions are adopting business practices to survive and

prosper. Principal investigators and top medical schools are not being forced into signing on with corporations. They are actively
courting the sponsorship of corporations because big companies
are usually the only ones with pockets deep enough to fund the
$500 million average cost of successfully developing a new drug.[78]
No one knows yet whether these partnerships will benefit patients
and medicine or damage the quality of scientific research.

One group of beneficiaries from the growth of CROs and
clinical research overall includes anyone who is looking for a job
at a CRO. A Web-based employment site in February 2007 listed
5,143 jobs with CROs.[79] An American Airlines in-flight magazine a year later carried a quarter-page ad for INC Research, a
CRO seeking to fill a wide range of positions including clinical
research associates, project managers, statistical programmers, and
clinical team leaders.[80]

In the past decade more than 150 educational institutions and
private companies have started to offer the specialized training
required for the fields of clinical trials research, management, and
execution.[81] The programs run the gamut from seminars and certificate courses to master's degrees and doctorates. Almost fifty
accredited academic institutions have full degree programs in clinical research. They include Harvard, the University of Michigan,
the University of Chicago, Johns Hopkins, and Duke University.[82]

One of the first academic programs was started in 1998 at
Durham Technical Community College, in the shadow of Duke
University and in the heart of a region with one of the largest
concentrations of companies devoted to clinical research in the
nation, with ninety pharmaceutical firms and CROs. Durham
Technical Community College's program was the brainchild of
an executive at Quintiles, the world's largest CRO, and the program continues to have a training partnership with Quintiles.[83]

Most of the people who enroll for an associate's degree or
certificate in clinical research at Durham Tech already hold a

four-year degree in chemistry, biology, or applied health, according Melissa Ockert, program director for the Clinical Trials Research Associate Program at Durham Tech. She says Tech graduates are required to take classes in bioethics and do extensive fieldwork as part of their education. The in-state tuition for the associate's program is about three thousand dollars, and starting salaries for graduates are in the low forty-thousand-dollar range. There is a waiting list each year to get into the program.[84]

In 2007, when Kansas and Missouri were aggressively wooing Quintiles to relocate, local and state governments in North Carolina persuaded them to stay in Durham with $25 million in economic incentives. Those tax breaks were part of an overall $60 million expansion by Quintiles that promised to add a thousand jobs with average salaries of sixty-five thousand dollars to Durham's local economy. The president of Quintiles says the company would have most certainly moved to another state if North Carolina hadn't come up with the incentives.[85]

In 2007 in Raleigh, North Carolina, INC Research received more than $14 million in state and local tax breaks and other givebacks for meeting a hiring goal of eleven hundred new jobs.[86] The only reported downside to all the new jobs being created at CROs was that it would produce "acute shortages" of qualified staff at local hospitals.[87]

A negative aspect of commercial clinical research is that profits can become a bigger consideration than finding answers to medical mysteries. In 1996 Nancy Olivieri, a hematologist from Toronto, Canada, discovered that a drug to treat an inherited blood disorder she was testing in a clinical trial at the Hospital for Sick Children carried unexpected risks. When she tried to inform subjects in the trial about what she discovered, Apotex, the drug company sponsoring the trial, threatened her with legal action, ostensibly because she had signed an agreement not to reveal Apotex's trade secrets. The company shut the trial down without disclosing the potential risk.[88]

A few months later Olivieri reviewed subject charts and found what she thought was another risk from the drug. Apotex again threatened to slap her with a lawsuit if she told the subjects or went public with her findings.[89] Olivieri turned to the hospital and to the University of Toronto, which she was affiliated with, for backing and for help. While both institutions paid lip service to protecting her academic freedom, they did not support her in her desire to go public.[90]

At the time this was happening, local governments across Canada were cutting their funding to universities and hospitals to ease a federal budget deficit. To make up for the lost funding, universities were aggressively courting corporations for donations. They apparently did a good job because many drug companies were preparing to donate millions of dollars to hospitals for "naming opportunities." Apotex preliminarily agreed to donate $20 million to the University of Toronto and $10 million to its affiliated hospitals. It was the largest such donation the university had ever received.

Though threatened with lawsuits and denied support from her hospital and her university, Olivieri went public with her concerns in 1998. Apotex and board members at the Hospital for Sick Children responded by going on the offensive and taking actions that came close to ending Olivieri's career before the Canadian Association of University Teachers, faculty members at the University of Toronto, and two experts in the blood disorder being studied by Olivieri in the clinical trial came to her defense. After independent investigations into the incident, Olivieri was exonerated of the accusations made by Hospital administrators against her.

The Constant Gardener by John le Carré was based in part on the Olivieri case. Other fallout from the incident included the

University of Toronto's revising its policy on clinical trials and how to manage other research sponsored by industry. The policy now states that researchers cannot be prevented from disclosing risks that come to their attention.

A report commissioned by the Canadian Association of University Teachers concluded that while settlements were reached in the Olivieri case, the issues it raised about the negative influence of corporate sponsorship on medical research and about how academic institutions were so quick to back a company over their own employee have not been "satisfactorily resolved across the country or elsewhere."[91]

There is no question that government agencies throughout the world and in the United States, most notably the FDA, have created in recent years new and tougher regulations governing clinical trials. Institutional review boards, which are composed of paid and volunteer physicians, administrators, and independent members of the community who oversee clinical trials and ensure they are carried out ethically, properly, and according to regulations are enjoying increased authority to do their work. An international standard known as Good Clinical Practice governs how to ethically carry out clinical trials from design to data reporting and has been widely adopted to provide guidance. But for the most part new regulations have succeeded only in creating an atmosphere of "simultaneous overregulation and underprotection."[92]

Even though IRBs have more authority, they are often too swamped monitoring regulations, procedures, and paperwork to protect subjects adequately.[93] They also have to monitor a higher number of trials. At the University of Virginia two IRBs made up of twenty-two full-time staff and volunteers monitor sixteen hundred biomedical trials and six hundred social/psychological trials. The boards meet once every two weeks.[94]

The range of activities that IRBs monitor has grown in com-

plexity and scope as clinical trials have become more complicated. They oversee grant applications, interviews with journalists, research design review, patient privacy complaints, and other
such workaday issues.[95] This intense focus on paperwork causes
tunnel vision on behalf of some members on IRBs so that they
become overly detail oriented, losing focus on the primary ob-
jective for which IRBs were created in 1979: the protection of
human research subjects.[96] The granularity can get silly at times.
A researcher, for instance, who was a decade into a clinical trial,
was asked by an IRB to take out the word "anemia" from a consent form for fear that potential subjects wouldn't understand what
it meant.[97]

The FDA doesn't seem to have a better handle than IRBs on
enforcing regulations meant to protect subjects. A report commissioned by the FDA in 2007 said the agency suffers from a
"plethora of inadequacies" that puts the "health of the population
of the U.S." at risk. The report also said that CROs fall through
the cracks of the existing regulations.

The report, conducted by the Office of the Inspector General
at the Department of Health and Human Services, excoriated the
FDA for its oversight of clinical trials. The report says the FDA did
not have an up-to-date system to even identify and build a database of all the clinical trials, clinical trials sites, and IRBs it was
charged with monitoring. It says the FDA inspects less than 1 percent of all trials. Out of the 350,000 trials sites the FDA had registered from 2000 to 2005 the agency inspected fewer than 3,000.
When a violation was discovered and the FDA sent out a warning
letter demanding corrective action take place, the agency more often than not didn't follow up to find out if the corrective action
was ever undertaken.[98]

Until existing legislation to monitor the safety of clinical trials is enforced, passing stricter laws is superfluous. Watchdog and

public interest groups are increasing their level of lobbying for legislation to hold companies and individuals who run and oversee the clinical trials industry more accountable. They are hitting companies where it hurts most, in their pocketbooks, but they are still a long way away from forcing significant reform.

Chapter 4

LEGAL TRIALS

O N AUGUST 25, 2002, fifty-two-year-old James "Butch" Quinn sat up abruptly in hospital bed number eighteen at Hahnemann University Hospital in Philadelphia, raised his arms above his head, tightened his fists, crossed his arms, and died.[1] He had actually already been dead for several seconds after his respirator and the experimental artificial heart in his chest had been disconnected; the spasm at the end was a typical involuntary movement common for patients when they are removed from life support.[2] That dramatic end typified the sad drama that surrounded Quinn's treatment as a subject in a clinical trial that resulted in a court case that resonates through the medical and legal worlds to this day.

Told that he had thirty days to live because of a failing heart, Quinn had volunteered to test an artificial heart that was manufactured by Abiomed.[3] Immediately after a ten-hour surgery to implant the heart, Quinn's lungs filled with fluid and he was placed on an oxygen machine.[4] The heart, however, performed up to expectations and in a few months the crisis not only passed, but Quinn was doing so well his caregivers at the hospital were running themselves ragged trying to keep pace with his improvement. A month later Quinn was introduced as a medical success story to the media at a press conference. Quinn told the reporters how he was thankful to be alive, grateful to enjoy God's blessings, and that he wanted to go home.[5]

Going home was postponed when less than a month later, on New Year's Eve, Quinn suffered a small stroke. Two weeks after that Quinn left the hospital and was moved to a nearby hotel as part of the transition to eventually getting him home. Medical equipment was installed in Quinn's two hotel rooms to replicate the intensive care unit at the hospital, but he was cared for mostly by doctors from Abiomed, the company sponsoring the clinical trial. He was not attended by any full-time physicians from the hospital nor did he receive round-the-clock professional care, a situation that infuriated Quinn's wife, Irene.

At the hotel Quinn's condition deteriorated until he was brought back to Hahnemann Hospital on February 3, when he was attached to a ventilator that helped relieve breathing problems that were plaguing him.

By this time Quinn and his wife were physically and mentally exhausted, and not just from the taxing ordeal of being a medical pioneer. Even though Hahnemann Hospital said they were sent by mistake, bills for Quinn's care kept arriving at the couple's home. In a single day Irene Quinn opened notices from collection agencies for more than thirteen thousand dollars in anesthesiology bills.[6] She had, by that time, quit her job to take care of her husband, who said he was in "excruciating pain" and still only wanted to go home. Doctors caring for him agreed that Quinn's treatment would be appropriate in a home setting because, they said, clinically they were not helping him much at the hospital.[7]

Having Quinn go home, though, was never part of Abiomed's or Hahnemann's plans. One person associated with the case says they worked hard to save Quinn's life—and succeeded—but had no provisions to care for him after he got well. "It was like, what do we do with him now?" Enabling Quinn to return to his house was made more difficult because Quinn lived in a house without air conditioning and the wiring wasn't sufficient to meet the energy requirements of sophisticated medical equipment or even to consistently maintain the power supply needed for the battery in his artificial heart. An Abiomed official admits they never made preparations for an extended home stay for Quinn because they did not expect subjects early in the trial to live long enough to go home. Because preparations for home health care had not been decided upon before the trial started, Abiomed and Hahnemann Hospital disagreed about which one of them would foot the bill for Quinn's follow-up care.[8] It took until August for Abiomed to say they would cover the costs, but only for a limited time.[9]

In March Irene Quinn suffered a nervous breakdown and was hospitalized for several days. By that time Quinn and his wife decided they needed legal representation because they felt neither the staff at the hospital nor officials from Abiomed were providing adequate care. After doing research on the Internet, Irene Quinn found several attorneys who might be qualified to take the case, including Alan Milstein. Described as the "king of the small but growing band of clinical trial attorneys,"[10] Milstein had successfully settled a lawsuit for an undisclosed sum against the University of Pennsylvania over the death of Jesse Gelsinger in a clinical trial. Irene Quinn told her husband about her research to find a lawyer and he said, "Either get me Johnnie Cochran or that Jewish guy from New Jersey who handed it to Penn."[11]

Milstein visited Quinn at his bedside and decided to take the case because for him it brought to the forefront all the ethical problems with clinical trials.[12] In late August Quinn suffered a major stroke. He was declared brain dead and removed from life support two days later. His widow, Irene, made sure that after the artificial heart was removed for study, her husband's heart was reimplanted into his body before his burial.[13]

After Quinn's death Milstein brought a lawsuit for damages against Hahnemann Hospital; Tenet HealthCare Corporation, the company that owns Hahnemann Hospital; Drexel University, the medical school affiliated with Hahnemann Hospital; Abiomed; and the patient advocate for the Quinns, a doctor who was paid by Abiomed for his services in the experiment.[14]

Milstein goes full-bore into each case, guns blazing, naming anybody even tangentially involved in any case where a clinical trial has risked or taken human life. That practice has drawn stern criticism, such as when he named the bioethicist Arthur Caplan as a defendant in the Gelsinger lawsuit against Penn. "It's terrifying," says Caplan, who spent ten thousand dollars in legal fees before being dropped from the suit. "This is not a good trend because research can prove risky no matter how careful you are in reviewing or monitoring it."[15]

Milstein is also not content to stay on the narrow legal path of pursuing cases on medical malpractice grounds. In an earlier case, he was representing subjects in a clinical trial testing a new cancer vaccine at the University of Oklahoma Health Sciences Center in Tulsa. The trial had been halted after an audit by the federal Office for Human Research Protection determined the institutional review board wasn't doing a thorough enough review and that the consent forms the subjects signed overstated the benefits and understated the risks of the trial.[16] Milstein said the actions by the IRB violated rights guaranteed under the U.S. Constitution for all people to be treated "with dignity."[17] Milstein's tactic of naming each member of the IRB in the lawsuit was without precedent and widened the scope of who can be held responsible for trials that go wrong.[18]

To the relief of IRB members throughout the country, a federal judge dismissed the lawsuit about a year after it was filed. Still, notice was effectively served that any and all parties involved in clinical trials were potential targets for litigation. Experts predicted that IRBs could start shying away from taking on clinical trials that looked the least bit risky. "If you're too careful, you get to the point where you start turning down research because there might be some bad publicity if it goes wrong," says Sanford Chodosh, M.D., head of Public Responsibility in Medicine and Research (PRIM&R) in Boston.[19] Milstein dismisses that concern and says the job of IRBs is to protect subjects, period, end of story.

Casting that wide a net in such a dramatic way is in keeping with Milstein's style and beliefs. He aspires to one day go before the Supreme Court and argue that the Nuremberg Code spelling out the rights of subjects in clinical trials is the proper basis for a new and enforceable U.S. law governing the ethics of clinical trials. That law would make the humane treatment of subjects unambiguous so that researchers and doctors either treat subjects properly or face charges for failing to do so.[20]

Milstein hasn't appeared before the Supreme Court yet, but he is getting a lot of attention and drawing notice to clinical trials as a new and emerging area of law. "This is something that never happened before," William Hirschhorn, director of the Office of Clinical Trials at Temple University School of Medicine in Philadelphia, says about a case Milstein brought against another prestigious cancer treatment center for how it handled two clinical trials. "Lawyers for the first time are seeing a lot of problems. Milstein opened the door for doctors to be held accountable."[21]

Even attorneys who may be on the other side of a case acknowledge that Milstein is bringing clinical trials out in the open as a legal specialty. Kendra Dimond, who represents researchers and research institutions for the Washington, D.C.-based law firm of Arent, Fox, Kintner, Plotkin & Kahn, puts it succinctly: "Alan has really hit a nerve."[22]

Milstein's arguments in the Quinn case were varied and compelling. They addressed a litany of issues and potential problems that make clinical trials extremely ripe targets for litigation. Even the recruitment of Quinn opened the clinical trial to litigation, according to Milstein, because telling Quinn he only had thirty

days to live and that the artificial heart was an opportunity to pro-
long his life was misleading. No pulmonologist can say with any
degree of certainty that a patient has thirty days to live, Milstein
contended.[23]

That brings up the legal issue of whether a person who is ill can
even give informed consent to participate in a clinical trial. Milstein is one attorney who thinks that terminally ill patients, for
example, are inherently incapable of giving informed consent because they are unduly motivated to receive therapy and not to participate for altruistic reasons in a clinical research study. Because
clinical trials are not therapy, because they are by definition research, terminally ill patients who do consent to participate in trials
are usually persuaded to do so because of therapeutic misconception, or the implication they will receive treatment in the trial.

For years clinical trials have hidden behind informed consent to
avoid and repel lawsuits. Arguments such as Milstein's and others'
challenging the wording and intention of informed consent have
started to wear away that armor and expose corporations and research institutions to lawsuits over clinical trials that never would
have been considered before. This is happening partly because
informed consent is not as straightforward as it once was. Two decades ago researchers only had to ensure that the subject was informed of the risks of the trial and consented to participate despite
those risks. Informed consent is now more multifaceted and complex, and the nuances require clarification in court, especially
when a subject is injured.

Suzanne Davenport, seventy-one, enrolled in a clinical trial at
UCLA to test a drug called Spheramine that would be implanted
into her brain to treat her Parkinson's disease. The former kinder-
garten teacher signed a consent form that said, among other
things: "If you are injured as a direct result of research procedures,
you will receive treatment at no cost. The University of California
does not provide any other form of compensation for injury."[24]

Similar compensation clauses have become common in consent forms to encourage subjects to enroll in trials.

After a series of initial tests at UCLA, and before Davenport received the implantation surgery, the operation was moved to Florida's Tampa General Hospital. The surgeon for the clinical trial was affiliated with the University of South Florida, and before the procedure Davenport signed another consent form with three injury clauses. The first clause said the University of South Florida would make financial damages available to Davenport if she received any injuries during the trial and if the injuries were caused by a university employee. Tampa General Hospital said in the second clause that the costs for treating any injury "may be the responsibility of you or your insurance company." The final clause, from Berlex, the company that developed the drug, said care would be provided at no cost to Davenport if the treatment required was "not ordinarily necessary for your condition."[25]

Following the surgery on January 14, 2005, it was immediately apparent that Davenport had serious problems. She couldn't sit up in a chair, she needed a diaper, and her mouth remained open constantly. In less than a year Davenport needed to be restrained in bed to keep from falling and she required round-the-clock care. While Medicaid paid for the majority of Davenport's stay in a nursing home, her family had to contribute seven hundred dollars per month and spent twenty-eight thousand dollars on her care. In the coming years medical costs for Davenport's care were projected to run into the millions. Her daughter sought compensation to cover the expected expenses and got opinions from doctors who thought Davenport's worsened condition was a direct result of the Spheramine and was not a result of the natural progression of her Parkinson's.[26]

However, officials involved with the trial thought maybe Davenport's condition was caused by her Parkinson's and wasn't a result of the clinical trial. That's when Davenport's daughter contacted a lawyer. In 2008 the case was still unresolved. No safety issues were reported from the commercial IRB overseeing the trial and late-stage testing of Spheramine was scheduled to start in 2009.[27]

Davenport's case may prove to be a template for other cases. A survey in the *New England Journal of Medicine* in 2007 found that only 16 percent of academic research institutions gave free care to subjects who were injured as a result of clinical trials. Figures aren't available on how many CROs and private companies provide free care for injury.[28]

Such issues, coupled with lax government oversights and IRBs that are either understaffed or ill equipped to handle the workload stemming from the increase in trials, appear to send the signal that lawyers need to get involved in clinical trials litigation to keep them safe and aboveboard. Lawyers are responding to that need by taking on clinical trials cases in increasing numbers. The Chubb Group of Insurance Companies and Ernst & Young, LLP, as far back as 2001, took enough notice of the increase that they held a seminar for professionals in the clinical trials industry telling them how they can be more ethical in their management of trials in order to avoid lawsuits.[29]

Some say that more lawyers, in particular personal injury lawyers, are taking on clinical trials cases just to make a buck. One lawyer said, "[T]here are huge stakes here. It involves pharmaceutical companies, biomedical research institutions—the amount of money involved is simply staggering."[30] Milstein takes strong exception to the idea that lawyers in clinical trials litigation are ambulance chasers. "That's such bullshit," he says. "The reason that there's more litigation is because more people are getting hurt in clinical trials. The reason more people are getting hurt in clinical trials is because there are more clinical trials."[31]

Even if the motivation for lawyers to become more involved in clinical trials isn't purely money, some say increased lawsuits will only stifle medical progress by making researchers more wary of undertaking trials. Others contend that the legal system doesn't move fast enough to address issues happening today. "Litigation certainly gets everyone's attention," says Robert M. Nelson, IRB chairman at Children's Hospital in Philadelphia, "but getting a monetary award eight years later doesn't do any good for changing practices at the time of the trial."[32]

In fact, there are instances when litigation has drawn attention to issues that spurred reform and improvements in short order. After Milstein's first clinical trials case, for the family of Jesse Gelsinger who died during a trial on gene therapy, the National Institutes of Health contacted all clinical trials investigators involved in gene therapy research and reminded them that deaths and adverse events in trials had to be reported to government regulators. The notice generated reports from eighty institutions about 652 adverse events. Seven of those adverse reports were deaths in experiments that hadn't been previously reported to the NIH. The reason they weren't reported was because the principal investigators and pharmaceutical companies sponsoring the trials considered such disclosures "confidential commercial information." Once aware of the scope of the problem, the NIH held a conflict of interest seminar for researchers involved in gene therapy and congressional hearings into gene therapy clinical trials soon followed.[33]

The field of litigation over clinical trials is relatively new, but it's developing rapidly. Milstein is pushing to have clinical trials litigation become a separate and new area of law. Right now clinical trials cases are tried as medical malpractice cases. But clinical trials are research, not medical treatment. Milstein says new guidelines and standards for trying clinical trials cases need to be established.

"I think there is ten to fifteen times as much research going on today as was going on in the 1970s," Milstein says. "It's even difficult to find out the true number of subjects in clinical trials.

But of course, if you wanted to find out how many mice are the subjects of experiments, you could find out to the mouse. If you want to find out how many monkeys there are, you can find out to the monkey. But you can't find out how many human beings are subjects. There's something wrong with that."[34]

Milstein makes a good living off the specialized work he does litigating clinical trials cases but he insists that's not his motivation for specializing in them. He says someone can make money and still do something good for mankind.

Others have echoed that sentiment, arguing it doesn't matter whether lawyers are out for money or whether they are crusaders for improvement as long as they help raise the standards of clinical trials. "Despite their greed and bad manners," Douglas R. Mackintosh, the president of a company that audits clinical trials, writes about clinical trials litigators, "they keep the game honest in an arena now teeming with clinical studies. You don't have to agree with their motives, or even their tactics. You just have to believe there should be a 'junkyard dog' cruising the streets ready to fight in your corner should all other protective mechanisms fail to ensure subject safety."[35]

Stephen DeCherney, M.D., an executive with the clinical research organization PRA International, disagrees, saying clinical trials standards are well maintained by free economy forces and that lawyers are counterproductive to ensuring subject safety. "[T]he market will punish a pharma company whose business practices are unethical," DeCherney says. "If the FDA delays the clearance of a new drug because of unreliable data, millions of dollars are lost for every day of delay. A firm may see its share value plummet as a result of the delays to which the stock market is exceptionally sensitive."[36]

Pharmaceutical companies and CROs have not been idly sitting by and relying only on the dynamics of the free market to protect their interests. Drug companies have filed cases in federal court claiming that if a drug approved by the FDA harms someone the company that made the drug cannot be sued. At least one such case has made it to the Supreme Court. The legal theory, called "pre-emption," says courts should not question the judgment of the FDA, which is the only agency qualified to make decisions about drugs, and once the FDA says a drug is safe, that should be the last legal word.

In one case, more than three thousand women brought a lawsuit against Johnson & Johnson claiming that the Ortho Evra estrogen patch caused strokes and heart attacks, and even killed forty women. Documents from Johnson & Johnson show that the company knew before the patch was sold that it released far more estrogen than was stated on the label. Even with test results in hand that revealed problems, it took six years for the company to change the label warning women about the true levels of estrogen in the patch. If courts rule in favor of pre-emption, such details wouldn't matter because courts wouldn't have the jurisdiction to hear such lawsuits.[37]

There is a recent precedent that makes it likely that pre-emption will become a legal standard that will have implications on clinical trials litigation for years to come. In early 2008 the Supreme Court ruled eight to one that Medtronic, a medical device manufacturer, couldn't be sued in state court for selling a faulty balloon catheter that injured a man. The suit couldn't move forward because the FDA had previously approved the device. The justices said that juries are not qualified to weigh evidence better than the FDA and so the FDA should not be second-guessed about its decision to approve the catheter. In their ruling the justices apparently agreed with the position of Medtronic's lawyer Theodore Olson, who said that "nothing is perfectly safe" and patients now and in the future would be more harmed than helped if the court ruled to "discourage the marketing of products that might save our lives."[38]

As these legal changes take place, and as they get reinterpreted and applied to clinical trials, it's likely that more lawyers will be going to court and taking on more and more cases, which Milstein says is not his ultimate goal. "Lenny Bruce once said if everything was perfect he would be in the unemployment line right behind Jonas Salk," Milstein says. "I would like to be there too."[39]

Chapter 5

THERE'S A SUBJECT BORN
EVERY MINUTE

INSTEAD OF LOOKING like a doctor's office, MDS Pharma Services' facility in Tempe, Arizona, is a clinical research organization that looks and operates like a factory.

The fifty-thousand-square-foot facility, at the South Mountain Commerce Center on Beautiful Lane, was expanded in 2002 to contain 120 beds. It has an intensive care unit that can accommodate up to twelve people at a time. It boasts an internal clinical laboratory and lush accommodations that rival those found at resorts. The site can house patients long term, even for months at a time, just like a hospital.[1] The enormous facility is owned and operated by a company that employs nearly four thousand people at thirty-nine research sites in twenty-six countries,[2] and it always has its doors open to anyone seeking to enroll in a clinical trial for money.

The first room one enters in the facility is a huge space with sixty or so chairs arranged five rows deep along the white cinder block walls. A hand-lettered sign in English and Spanish tells potential subjects to wait for their name to be called at the time of their appointment. On a chilly January morning the subjects waiting to be screened to test a new drug for epilepsy are overwhelmingly Hispanic; there are a few Native Americans and even fewer white people. Most are healthy working-class men and women; some are students. Before each of them arrives at MDS for a physical examination they fill out a health questionnaire on the Internet. They then answer more in-depth health questions, such as family medical history, on the phone. If they pass those screenings, they're invited to come to the medical facility for further screening.[3]

When their names are called they go in small groups to have their IDs checked and logged in to confirm the birthdates, addresses, and Social Security numbers they provided on the Internet form. At this stage of the process the halls of the facility seem as busy as the four lanes of traffic less than a mile away on Interstate 10. Nurses question potential subjects in Spanish and English to sort out the logistics for each. They then hand each person a packet of information with the words "Together, we're making lives better" in big letters on the top page. They are told they should read the literature while they wait to meet with a nurse to discuss and sign the consent form.

The packet contains a schedule for the clinical trial. The timeline is exhaustive. It accounts for each and every minute of the four nights and three days the subjects will be housed in the facility testing the new drug:

- 7:50 A.M.—Vital signs
- 7:55 A.M.—Blood draw
- 8:00 A.M.—No lying down—Start water restriction
- 8:15 A.M.—Blood draw[4]

The packet also contains general instructions on what not to eat or drink before and during the trial; a nine-page consent form; important phone numbers; a list of expectations and responsibilities for each subject; and, most important for most of those seeking to enroll, information on how subjects receive payment.[5]

Down a hall there are half a dozen small rooms where the subjects go in groups to have the consent form explained to them and have any questions answered. In one room a Native American who looks to be in his mid-forties, an African-American college student, and a white, unemployed man in his early forties listen to a nurse explain the clinical trial. It's a Phase I study for an epilepsy drug that has never been marketed before. Previously, eight groups of healthy men took the drug. As with all Phase I studies, each group took higher and higher doses to determine the physical and emotional effects and side effects of the increased dosages on healthy people before the next phase of testing on subjects with the condition.

"Everyone walked out on their own two feet," the nurse says about the previous study subjects.

"That's a relief," one potential subject says.[6]

The nurse goes on to tell the fifty-four subjects in the study that they will receive either the experimental drug or a placebo during the clinical trial. She explains to the subjects that blood will be drawn up to nineteen times during the three days they are at MDS. Urine samples will be taken throughout the study and sometimes in the middle of the night to check each subject's general health and determine if he or she has signs of alcohol or drug abuse. Each subject will have sixteen electrocardiograms during the study. The nurse tells them the FDA is asking for more cardiac monitoring in clinical trials since heart attacks showed up as a side effect of Vioxx only after it was on the market.[7] Possible side effects from the experimental epilepsy drug include "headache, numbing sensation in the back of the mouth, a metallic taste, dry throat, anxiety, shivering, and palpitations."[8]

At this point the nurse asks if there are any questions. There are none. Then she goes over the section about how much money each subject will be paid for taking part in the trial.

The amount to be paid depends on how much of the study each subject completes. If a subject completes the entire study, which includes the three-day confinement and two return visits, they will be paid $830. If the subject only completes the three-day confinement, they are paid $584.[9]

At that point there is a question: Is there a penalty if a subject leaves early? The nurse says that will be determined on a case-by-case basis.

The nurse then has each subject read aloud from the consent form to make sure the all can read. Each subject then initials and signs the nine-page form. From there they go through a series of physical examinations similar to what army recruits go through on induction day. Lines form and each subject waits his or her turn to have their height, weight, blood pressure, and electrocardiograms logged. They then have their blood drawn and see a doctor who looks down their throats, has them follow a light with their eyes, and checks their pulse.

The whole screening process, from walking through the front door at MDS to going back out to the parking lot with a copy of the consent form and the informational packet in hand, takes about two hours. It is handled as briskly and professionally as any common business transaction. And that's exactly what it is, a business deal between a multinational company and people who want to make money off participating in clinical trials.

Subjects who label themselves "guinea pigs" sign up for clinical trials for money and oftentimes are treated like the hired help. In 1938 gastroenterologist William Osler Abbott, M.D., undertook a series of clinical trials that aided in the eventual creation of the Miller-Abbott tube, a four-yard length of hollow plastic swallowed by patients to help diagnose and treat intestinal and stomach ailments. The methods Dr. Abbott used to achieve this significant medical advance, however, reveal how little researchers sometimes think of paid test subjects.

He bypassed the idea of using dogs to swallow the tube, which had an inflated balloon at one end enabling radiated fluoroscopes (an early progenitor of x-rays) to be taken because he considered animal testing a "waste of time."[10] He preferred going straight to testing on human subjects. When Dr. Abbott, an instructor at the hospital at the University of Pennsylvania, couldn't find patients there willing to volunteer for his experiment, he decided to pay subjects to participate. Finding healthy people willing to swallow his four-yard-long experimental invention wasn't easy. An unemployment agency refused to even advertise for subjects when they heard what they had to test. Dr. Abbott had people hand out leaflets that said subjects would be paid two dollars per day. Even in the hardest days of the Great Depression, there were no takers. Then Dr. Abbott was told about Henry, a black janitor at the hospital, who might be able to solve his subject shortage. Abbott paid Henry fifty cents for every subject he recruited. He brought in so many that soon subjects were literally lined up every morning at eight thirty outside the lab door and additional subjects were scheduled for tests weeks in advance.

The subjects, though healthy, were not always to Abbott's liking. "I'm sure my animals had a larger intake of corn liquor, pork chops and chewing tobacco than the white rats in the medical school, but at least they're human," Abbott told an audience of doctors in New York in 1939 when he recounted his clinical trials experience with the Miller-Abbott tube. The topic of his presentation that day, to eminently renowned physicians and researchers who were members of the Charaka Club, was unambiguously titled "The Problem with the Professional Guinea Pig."[11]

Abbott complained that one time Henry "slipped in an epileptic" who bit off the end of the tube during a seizure. Luckily, Abbott reported, he was able to retrieve the tube from the subject with no harm to the experiment. When one subject named Jim was found during a test to have a bullet lodged near his spine because his lover had recently shot him for being seen out earlier that day with another woman, Abbott despaired about his plight—his own, not the subject's. "Such events led me at times to wish I could keep my animals in metabolism cages," Abbott said. He was also irked when subjects took pens and inkwells from the hospital dispensary.[12]

Despite the distaste Abbott had for his subjects, they were crucial in helping him perfect his advanced diagnostic tool. Things were going so well that by 1935 Abbott prepared to present the tube to the annual convention of the American Medical Association in Atlantic City. For his presentation he needed two subjects per day for each of the four days he was going to show off his new invention at the meeting. He promised a "liberal bonus" to the men who agreed to take part. The problem was that none of the men would. Abbott's subjects, perhaps thinking less of him than he thought of them and knowing they had the doctor in a delicate spot, went on strike, demanding double the pay they were receiving.

Dr. Abbott would have none of it. In a desperate move he went into classes at the University of Pennsylvania and pleaded for students to volunteer so he could make his presentation. Not completely trusting in the altruism of the students to submit themselves to uncomfortable tests for the benefit of medicine alone, he offered them the same daily rate he was paying his subjects before the walkout. It worked. After promptly rounding up enough student "volunteers," Dr. Abbott fired his entire group of paid subjects. His presentation, "Exhibit of the Small Intestine," won Abbott a special certificate of honor from the AMA.[13]

Enrolling in a clinical trial for money is not a recognized profession; human guinea pigs can't strike en masse for better wages, for instance. But with an untold number of subjects being paid up to and above seventy-five hundred dollars[14] for undergoing all sorts of pharmaceutical and medical tests, it is a way that a lot of people these days are making money. (According to a 1996 article in the *Wall Street Journal*, forty thousand healthy subjects

were enrolled in Phase I clinical trials. While that number has not been updated by a reputable source since then, some estimate there are one hundred thousand human guinea pigs now working.) The practice has been given a name by those who take part in it: "guinea-pigging."[15] They even share their own lingo: Being housed during a long-term study is called a "lockdown." A "washout" is the name for the month-long, mandatory waiting period between clinical trials that guinea pigs go through to get all the drugs they ingested from the previous testing out of their systems.[16]

The number of guinea-piggers has been growing in recent years. With patient recruitment the most challenging and time-consuming part of clinical trials, the money paid to test subjects has increased, making it a more lucrative proposition and attracting more subjects.[17] But who exactly are these people?

In the 1960s paid guinea-piggers didn't exist. Companies usually estimated dosages for new medications, and researchers would give out drugs to doctors their drug representatives knew, asking them to try them out on patients. When thalidomide caused birth defects in pregnant European women in 1962 the U.S. Congress passed laws to keep the same sort of medical nightmare from befalling the American public. When laws mandated the FDA to oversee drug testing on animals and on healthy people in Phase I clinical trials to determine the maximum dose of any new drug that can be delivered before the medication becomes harmful or toxic, pharmaceutical companies went into jails searching for prisoner/subjects to test new drugs. They recruited so many inmates that soon almost all Phase I clinical drug trials were being conducted behind prison walls. But in the mid-1970s there was enough of a public outcry over the practice of using poverty-stricken prisoners as guinea pigs (and often giving the prisoners early parole in exchange for signing on to participate in the research) that the FDA mandated that all subjects had to give voluntary informed consent that was free from coercion, such as a promise of early parole. The new FDA regulations didn't forbid using prisoners, but drug companies stopped the practice anyway.[18]

In 1974 the pool of readily available guinea pigs dried up when reports of the Tuskegee experiments became widely known, making volunteering for clinical trials a decidedly unsavory proposition in the public mind. Money then became an effective enticement for healthy subjects to join Phase I clinical trials. Drug companies, working through CROs and universities, set up clinics, took out ads, and started writing checks. One drug company, Eli Lilly, had had a clinic open in Indianapolis since 1926. In the 1970s Lilly's board members and business executives endorsed a practice, approved by an independent board that ran the clinic, of recruiting homeless people as subjects in clinical trials. The company viewed the exploitive practice as a humanitarian act. They figured while they were taking part in long-term clinical trials the subjects were, at least for a little while, removed from the danger of living on the street and provided with hot meals, warm beds, medical care, and time to detox from drugs and alcohol.

"Test subjects welcome the free physical exams and the money they get," a Lilly executive said to the *Wall Street Journal* in 1996 when the paper did an exposé on Lilly's practice of aggressively recruiting homeless subjects at the Indianapolis clinic. They are, the executive insisted, motivated "by altruism . . . These individuals want to help society."[19]

In addition to "helping society," subjects left the Lilly clinic packing a big wad of cash—sometimes more than four thousand dollars—made from withstanding multiday, in-house studies.[20] In return for their largesse, Lilly was supplied with a population of poor subjects in desperate need of cash. It seemed like a win-win situation except for a few flaws. For instance, since most of the subjects were alcoholics, were they capable of giving non-coerced, informed consent when money was dangled in front of them to sign up to be subjects?

While such questions about the ethicality of Lilly's practices in Indianapolis went unasked and unanswered, the reputation of the clinic spread like wildfire, attracting homeless alcoholics from across the country to its doors and beds. One subject, a former crack addict and still an alcoholic who heard about the clinic in Nashville, Tennessee, said he was signing up for a trial so he could get enough money to buy a car and some shoes. Another subject, Joseph LaDuke, didn't get to make any such investments. He left the Lilly clinic flush with more than two thousand dollars and immediately hit the bars. After a few drinks he outfitted himself in a new pair of Nikes, some new jeans, and a new shirt. He didn't hang on to the clothes for all that long, though. LaDuke blacked out before midnight and woke up in jail with no clothes on and no bankroll, which he believes his drinking buddies relieved him of so they could party on their own. The only things he ended up with were the Nikes and charges for public drinking and disorderly conduct. LaDuke was not left completely high and dry without resources. After doing his jail time, LaDuke called the Lilly clinic. Early on a Monday morning he was let into the facility by a Pinkerton guard, ready to sign up as a subject in another clinical trial.[21]

In addition to raising the ire of those who advocate for better treatment of subjects in clinical trials, such stories raise the questions of whether subjects can be harmed by the drugs they're taking and whether the results of testing on such people as LaDuke produce trustworthy results. Roger Wilkins, from the FDA's Center for Drug Evaluation and Research, told the *Wall Street Journal* in 1996 that testing on alcoholics means if something goes wrong and a subject isn't feeling well it's hard to say whether it's from the drug being tested or from alcoholism or alcohol withdrawal. Other doctors contend that drugs are metabolized differently in a drinker than in a nondrinker and the difference can alter test results. Another doctor says that testing on alcoholics compromises the efficiency of the testing and jeopardizes the very safety of the drugs being tested.[22] Despite these concerns, a former official at Lilly says it was "no secret" that many of the subjects at their Indianapolis clinic were homeless alcoholics. In 1996 an official at Lilly disagreed and said previous alcohol use had no effect on trial results and that current use would be uncovered during the pre-screening process.[23]

It isn't as if the subjects at the Lilly clinic showed up for their screenings loaded to the gills on Mad Dog 20/20. Most homeless subjects were well versed on how to detox enough so they would pass the screening and become eligible for studies. They spent the days before their screenings drinking herbal tea, oil, or vinegar or eating raisins, liver, and other iron-rich foods to scrub their bodies and organs free of booze. Some even quit drinking for up to ten days in order to gain admittance. Even if they only did a so-so job of sobering up, the homeless were still accepted as subjects with a wink and a nod because, as one Lilly official says, as long as they were sober at the time of their screening, they were usually recruited.[24]

The way the Lilly clinic operated in 1996 was considered emblematic of the methods many drug companies and CROs used when they were recruiting subjects. An FDA official at the time said he had not seen anything that made the practices at the Lilly clinic seem any worse or better than practices taking place at other clinical trials. "But," he said, "we haven't looked."[25]

Nine years later, in 2005, a CRO was accused of enrolling undocumented immigrants in clinical trials to test drugs at a shabby, five-story converted Holiday Inn in Miami. The building wasn't just some little clinic run by a small company, either. The 675-bed site was the largest clinical trials site in the United States. It was owned and run by SFBC International (now called Pharmanet

Development Group), one of the largest CROs in the world at the time. The site's rooms had scuffed walls and floors, bathrooms with chipped tiles that reeked of urine, and waiting rooms jammed with undocumented aliens. Many of the potential subjects didn't understand the confusing language in the consent forms and were only there because they were being paid.[26] One forty-one-year-old from Venezuela was waiting to be a subject only because he needed money to send to his family back home.[27] Side effects from the drug he was testing to get that money were not the only risks the subject faced.

The director of SFBC's medical trials in 2005, Lisa Krinsky, got her medical degree from a Caribbean medical school and was not licensed to practice medicine in the United States.[28] But Krinsky wasn't the only unlicensed clinician working in clinical trials. FDA records revealed that quite a few of the fifteen thousand clinics running trials use unlicensed clinicians in studies. The exact number of how many were unlicensed was difficult to come by because many of the centers keep poor records. What records are available show that the people who perform up to 90 percent of the hands-on testing in some trials use staff, relatives, and sometimes even themselves to test drugs. An official from the FDA says it's not uncommon for the staff providing most of the person-to-person care in clinical trials to have no qualifications at all, or to have gone to a one-day seminar that allowed them to be called "certified" study coordinators.[29]

The lapse in Krinsky's credentials went overlooked by the institutional review board responsible for independently monitoring SFBC's clinical trials. One reason for that may have been because the commercial IRB hired to monitor the safety of SFBC's trial was owned by the wife of SFBC's vice president of clinical operations.

That kind of coziness is one example of the frequently close relationships that develop—a closeness that some say is motivated by profits—between supposedly independent IRBs and corporate sponsors of clinical trials. One bioethicist said trusting commercial, for-profit IRBs gave him "hives" because he'd never "seen an IRB advertise by saying, 'Hire us. We're the most zealous enforcer of regulations you could have.' People say, 'We'll turn it around faster. We're efficient. We know how to get you to your deadline.' "[30]

After the disturbing news about the poor conditions and questionable recruiting practices in SFBC's Florida facility became public, the company hired two independent law firms to review the allegations. SFBC's directors said the report exonerated the company.[31] Even though they were exonerated, they demolished the facility in May 2006 and in 2007 paid out $28.5 million to settle a class-action lawsuit related to their treatment of subjects.[32] That sounds like a large settlement but shrinks in light of the company's 2005 revenues of more than $300 million.[33]

Many human guinea pigs are neither drunks nor illegal immigrants. Typical clinical trials' subjects in the United States, whether enrolled for pay or for more altruistic reasons, are white men in their mid-forties who earn less pay and have less education than the average American male.[34] Some insist that that demographic is very generous in describing the kinds of people who really sign up to be guinea pigs. University of Minnesota bioethicist Carl Elliott writes in the *New Yorker*, "Because such studies require a fair amount of time in a research unit, the subjects are usually people who need money and have a lot of time to spare: the unemployed, college students, contract workers, ex-cons, or young people living on the margins who have decided that testing drugs is better than punching a clock with the wage slaves."[35]

Motivated by the paycheck waiting at the end of their trial, some subjects naturally stretch the truth about whether they really meet the criteria demanded by the researchers of the study. For the clinical trial at MDS Pharma Services that paid $830, much of the information from potential subjects was taken on good faith alone and was not medically verified. For that particular trial, restrictions on subjects included that they not smoke or chew tobacco or put nicotine in their body six months before the start of the study; they not take any over-the-counter drugs for fourteen days before check-in for the study; that they refrain from taking any drugs that can alter liver or kidney clearance for thirty days before check-in; and that they not take any prescription drugs for fourteen days before check-in.[36] The blood and urine tests screened for hepatitis B and C, HIV, and cotinine, a by-product of nicotine and tobacco.[37] One subject who passed the blood and urine screening and physical examination and was invited to participate in the study was at the time taking prescription antibiotics and the painkillers Vicodin and Percocet for nine days for a toothache. He was also on Wellbutrin, Vytorin, and the high blood pressure medication Liprosil for two months before the screening.[38] The motivation for the subject to be less than truthful about violating these restrictions is obvious: $830.

A gastrointestinal trial at a university lab in Philadelphia required the paid subjects to stay on a very restricted diet during a five-week hospital stay. One study participant, however, says the diet was making the subjects crazy with hunger. They were starving so much that one night they broke into a food storage area to chow down on cookies and Cheez Doodles. The extracurricular snacking may have jeopardized the subjects' health and definitely skewed the results of the trial.[39]

Nicholas Pesa doesn't fit the typical guinea pig profile. He is a twenty-six-year-old med student at Case Western University who, in his four-year career as a guinea pig, made ten thousand dollars donating sperm and three hundred dollars for providing a biopsy from inside his lung. The lung procedure wasn't nearly as pleasant an experience as donating sperm. "I didn't think it was going to hurt as much as it did," Pesa says. "For a good couple of days afterward, it really sucked."[40]

It didn't suck enough to stop him from enrolling in clinical trials, however. Even after the painful lung procedure, Pesa remains a member in good standing of the Guinea Pig Gang, a loose affiliation of Cleveland medical school students who enroll in trials for cash. They only enroll in a study, however, if it meets specific criteria.

The four rules that Guinea Pig Gang members Pesa, Jason Snyder, and Nikolai Sopko drew up and adhere loosely to are: There has to be a low risk of the trial causing long-lasting damage; the money they're paid has to be decent, at least better than getting just five dollars for having their blood drawn; they have to know before the trial what kind of painkillers, if any, they will be given; and the trial has to be sponsored by a trustworthy research institution. (Although Sopko admits that if the first three rules are in place, he would let the fourth rule slide.)[41]

When selecting studies to take part in, guinea-piggers appear to consider comfort (or its close cousin, safety) and money first and last. For his first clinical trial, a subject known as "Guinea Pig J," answered a newspaper ad recruiting subjects and spent four weekends testing a generic drug. Looking back six years later, after he had tested heart medications and drugs to treat Parkinson's along with a host of other generic drugs and had become more of a savvy pro at guinea-pigging, J admits there was a serious problem with his first trial. He only got five hundred dollars, or about eight dollars per hour. "I realize now that was a terrible study," J says. "I rank studies on the number of days per cash you get."[42]

As far as safety, before each trial begins J gets a manila folder describing the possible side effects of what he is testing and that helps him make up his mind; he won't sign up for a study where the "side effects get too crazy."

J considers most clinical trials—those conducted by reputable companies or hospitals—safe. "You just have to trust the company," he says. "This is really pretty mainstream."[43]

Whether a guinea-pigger is as trusting as J, or whether one is prone to research every aspect of the trial they'll be signing up for, they share something in common with members of the Guinea Pig Gang. They have to employ their wits and networking skills to make sure they are going into the best paying, most comfortable, and safest studies. They frequently rely on word of mouth or stick with recruiters from institutions they know and trust. The Internet though is increasingly becoming the water cooler where guinea-piggers are able to gather and share information about the safety and comfort offered in past or future clinical trials, swap war stories, and get the scoop on their profession.

Paul Clough is a twenty-eight-year-old guinea-pigger who also created a guinea pig Web site. He figures getting information about trials on the Web is better than how he heard about his first study, which was from a homeless guy who told him about guinea-pigging when Clough said he needed work. In 2004 Clough moved to Austin, Texas, and it wasn't to enjoy the music scene. It was because he heard through the guinea pig grapevine that Austin had a large concentration of CROs and universities testing drugs and procedures for pharmaceutical companies. Another such hub drawing guinea pigs includes the Raleigh-Durham region in North Carolina. The Philadelphia area is home to so many research institutions, CROs, and pharmaceutical companies that guinea pigs commonly refer to it as "pharm country."[44] Clough's CRO of choice for trials is PPD, Pharmaceutical Product Development, which he says does up to four thousand clinical trials a year. Such tidbits are all available on his Web site, guineapigsgetpaid.net, which is a comprehensive information source where Clough shares his good fortune of making up to twenty-eight thousand dollars per year being a guinea pig.[45]

The site's frequently asked questions page answers and

addresses just about any concern a potential guinea pig might have, from the nuts and bolts logistics such as needing to have a Social Security number to enroll in a trial to more ephemeral topics like being polite and presenting a good appearance during the screening or during a lockdown. If you're wondering how soon prior to the screening for a trial you should stop drinking alcohol, the site tells you. (In case you're curious, enjoy your last binge at least one week before a trial. If you go on the wagon one week or sooner before the screening your liver enzymes might be messed up and you'll be rejected.) If you're worried about what kind of guinea-piggers you might be bunking with during your trial, the site can help you out. It tells you all about dealing with guinea-piggers from the "Jerry Springer crowd," meaning unsavory characters who might be homeless or drug addicted. It also wisely advises not to believe the tall tales told by veteran guinea-piggers about prior trials, such as having a toe cut off and sewed back on.[46]

Although Clough is more afraid of getting hit by a drunk driver than he is of getting harmed in a clinical trial, he says that research about clinical trials is a key requirement if you're going to be a guinea-pigger and the Web site helps fulfill that need for knowledge. Aside from making him a little money, Clough hopes his site will help human guinea pigs stay safe by raising their awareness of what they are getting into. "It's up to the [subjects] to be honest during the evaluation process to avoid being hurt," Clough says. "The whole process is based on mutual trust, but to do it safely, you have to be well informed."[47]

A forty-eight-year-old woman guinea-pigger who lives in North Carolina endorses Clough's position. The mother of three children is an EMT who is married to a guy who works in a lumberyard. She has held jobs as a temp worker, a substitute teacher, a factory worker, a home health technician, and now as a guinea pig who does up to five trials a year. She enjoys the people she meets during trials, such as at one weekend study when she roomed with a model, a doctor, a woman once married to a millionaire, and a student. She likes how learning about new medical advancements informs her training as an EMT.

During her "career" she has been through several MRIs, had a chunk of her right thigh removed for testing, and had more blood drawn than she can remember. Despite all that, she bristles at the notion that she is some sort of victim who is taken advantage of because she is a guinea pig. "When you sign that consent form you're saying I am responsible even if my insides fall out," she explains. "And you know if you want to do the next study you have to stay good and healthy. It keeps you on your toes."[48]

Some guinea pigs simply trust market forces to keep them safe. They figure it's just not in the interest of a big pharmaceutical company or CRO to injure or kill a subject.[49] This Adam Smith approach to safely making it through a medical experiment doesn't guarantee positive results. A nineteen-year-old student killed herself in 2004 after testing the antidepressant Cymbalta. In a clinical trial in Montreal one man was in a bed next to another subject who was coughing up blood. He asked to be moved but remained where he was. Later he and eight other subjects in the trial contracted tuberculosis.[50]

The three members of the Guinea Pig Gang understand the medical risks of each procedure they put themselves through better than the average guinea pig because they're medical students. However, their youth leads them to take risks occasionally that the average guinea pig wouldn't consider. As Pesa went through the consent process before his lung biopsy he was only half listening, preferring instead to concentrate more intently on an upcoming workout than on the risks that were being listed. When the research assistant told him that one patient had died during the trial, Pesa forgot about his gym date and paid much closer attention to what he was getting into. He considered dropping out but they were paying $300, an amount of cash that to him sounded too good to pass up. Pesa went ahead. He spent the next couple of days in pain, but he lived.[51]

Not all healthy guinea pigs who sign up for trials are as lucky as Pesa. A healthy seventy-year-old nurse named Elaine Holden-Able who signed up to test the dietary supplement methionine died from an overdose of the supplement. The trial was conducted by a researcher at Case Western University and paid for with money left over from an Alzheimer's study sponsored by a tobacco company in 2001. An autopsy showed that Holden-Able had ten times the normal level of methionine in her system.[52] The hospital investigated the death and labeled it a "tragic human accident."[53]

Following the hospital's internal review, the Office for Human Research Protection, which oversees all clinical trials that receive government funding, investigated Holden-Able's death.[54] The agency was at a disadvantage even before their investigation began because officials at Case Western didn't inform OHRP about the "adverse event" until four months after Holden-Able died. OHRP officials didn't even travel from Washington, D.C., to Cleveland to interview people involved in the clinical trial. Instead, OHRP investigators reviewed the hospital's own internal report on the death, found no fault, and ended their investigation with no penalties against the hospital.[55]

In Holden-Able's case there at least was an investigation, which is a rare occurrence in the world of clinical trials. While the FDA inspects about 1 percent of all clinical trials,[56] the OHRP investigates less than 1 percent of the adverse events in trials reported voluntarily by academic research institutions.[57] It wasn't until 2005 that the FDA even designated a numeric code that inspectors could fill in on forms to report "failure to protect the rights, safety, and welfare of subjects."[58]

Guinea-piggers deliberately put themselves at greater risk than average clinical trials subjects because more risk equals more money. The more invasive and uncomfortable the procedure, the more subjects get paid.[59] Also, the more time a trial takes the more they're paid. Some trials requiring subjects remain in a facility for up to several weeks or even months are jackpots.

So, what do subjects stuck in a medical facility getting poked and prodded while studying drugs and procedures *do* all day long? Lucky ones are housed in swank facilities that are more like vacation destinations than laboratories. The better clinical trials sites have TV, wireless Internet, video games, quiet rooms, and movies. "It was like a hotel," says one trial subject who was housed in a private room with a TV during his multiday stay, "except that twice they came in and stuck a tube down my throat."[60]

But some trials that don't require lockdowns can not only be exhausting, they can be thoroughly dehumanizing, a reminder that as a guinea pig you are just a hired, nameless cog in a medical experiment. One subject who signed up for a trial to identify brain markers in schizophrenics discovered that eighteen hours of psychological testing was anything but "noninvasive." Instead it was invasive in a way that was more insidious than if someone had stuck a tube down his throat. The trial, which did not involve taking drugs, consisted of answering questions and playing games in clinical interviews, brainwave testing, an eye movement exam, and other neuropsychological examinations. The pay was eleven dollars per hour plus a voucher for lunch served at the 1700s-era Spring Grove Psychiatric Hospital, where the tests were conducted.[61]

The subject, Mikita Brottman, spent the first few hours on a part of the hospital campus that in 1917 was called the Psychopathic Building, answering a battery of yes or no questions. Then he went to have the neuropsych exam. As fancy as the exam sounded to him, it ended up that he simply played with ancient toys and games while a researcher made notes; took memory word tests where he had to repeat details of stories just read to him;

spoke into a tape recorder and related the story of Cinderella; gave his opinion about why people believe in God; and used his finger to trace lines on a piece of paper.

It was hours later, at about six in the evening, when the final test for the day was done. It involved watching a series of symbols on a computer then clicking on a mouse to predict where the next symbol should be. A bell went off and Brottman would win ten cents if he got the answer right. If he got it wrong a buzzer would go off and he lost a dime. For his efforts Brottman got a headache and a little more than two dollars. Because the first day of testing was so unexpectedly exhausting and boring, it took a lot for Brottman to go back for the second day of tests two weeks later, but he did.[62]

He was put in a laboratory and electrodes were attached to his head to measure his brainwaves in response to a series of audible tones that were played. His responses to hearing buzzing noises were also measured. Again, it went on for several mind-numbing hours.

The next and last test took place in the eye lab and, to Brottman, became more like a scene in *A Clockwork Orange*—the one in which researchers reprogram Malcolm McDowell's criminal brain by strapping him down, forcing his eyes open so he can't blink, and making him watch a screen flooded with imagery designed to remove all his sociopathic impulses. At first Brottman looked through two pinholes and followed dots with his eyes. Then he had to look through the pinholes and not blink—exactly like the character in *A Clockwork Orange*. Brottman was one of about seven hundred subjects to have gone through the trial, which explains to him why most of the researchers seemed so lackadaisical and uninspired while they were administering the tests. By the end of the testing Brottman was keenly aware of his value—or lack thereof—as a person as opposed to his value as a test subject. "All that was needed from me, essentially, was good data," Brottman writes. "Of course, this is what guinea pigs are for—but since these were psychological experiments, I'd hoped the researchers would be more interested in my mind than my brain. In the end, however, I realized that, like most other employees, what they were mainly interested in was what they'd be doing when they got out of work at five."

Brottman was paid about two hundred dollars for the study.[63]

Even pulling a lockdown in an upper echelon clinic doesn't change the fact that guinea-pigging is a really boring way to make a living; more like having to endure a stay in a hospital when you're not even sick than enjoying a cool getaway.

One subject, identified only as #1J, thought she hit it big when she was approved for a twenty-two-night/twenty-three-day clinical trial. The thirty-three hundred dollars she would be paid was only one highpoint. The study required no food or water restrictions, there would not be too many blood draws, and the drugs she was testing had already been approved by the FDA. The downside was that the two approved drugs were being studied to see how they interacted. And they were mind-altering drugs for treating depression, schizophrenia, and bipolar disorder.

On the second day of the study #1J woke up at eight forty-five A.M., took a dose of Lexapro, wrote some letters, read, and had lunch. So far so good. Then she went to sleep until the afternoon because the Lexapro zonked her out completely. In two days #1J had read two books and five magazines. The highlight of her stay up to that point was that they served chicken strips for dinner on the second night. By day five #1J settles into her routine: "Dose, eat breakfast, nap, eat lunch, nap, read, write, eat dinner, shower, read, eat snack, go to bed." Throughout the study she plays board games with her fellow subjects, gets occasional visitors, goes for short walks, and sits looking out the window in the lounge. She also goes nearly out of her mind from boredom.

As the study wears on, they start mixing Lexapro with another drug to see what happens. For #1J the worst side effect is sleepiness. Things are tougher for her fellow guinea pigs. Many of them can't sleep at all. Others become jittery; they have muscle spasms and trouble concentrating, and they experience weird changes in their thinking patterns. One subject wonders out loud why the sponsor doesn't just end the trial and put "us out of our misery."

On day twenty-three it comes to an end, and #1J leaves with few worries because she's been told the drugs shouldn't cause withdrawal symptoms once she's off them. After one last blood draw that goes badly because they have to access a small vein and it takes a long time, #1J gets her "honorarium" check, goes to IHOP with friends to have pumpkin pancakes, goes to a store to get some beer, then hangs out at a strip mall where she enjoys being thirty-three hundred dollars richer. She also leaves the study pleased that because she was such a good subject, they will consider her for other clinical trials.[64] As boring and potentially risky as the clinical trial was for #1J, it holds out the exciting prospect of a career as a guinea pig.

Bob Helms knows all about the underworld of people who have careers as guinea pigs. He's been called a "pioneer in the world of guinea-pig activism"[65] who believes the ad hoc work should be treated as a recognized trade. Belying his former career as a union organizer, Helms advocates strongly for guinea pigs to enjoy regulated working conditions, benefits, and the kinds of rights extended to people in other "professions."

Helms, who is fifty-one, has put himself through about ninety clinical trials for the money. He only stopped when he turned forty-five, which is a common cutoff age for healthy subjects enrolling in trials. He is the founder of a magazine and Web site called *Guinea Pig Zero*, which he started to mark the sixtieth anniversary of the Nuremberg Trials. The site provides advice and information to people enrolling in trials for money. (The Web site still operates, while the magazine printed its last issue in 2000.)

He got his start in the guinea pig business in 1995 when he was working as a union organizer at a hospital. He knew dozens of people, mostly artists and political activists, who were making money by signing up for trials. They told him it was good work, so he jumped on board to make a little extra cash. "Little" was the operative word. For Helms, unlike for others, guinea-pigging didn't bring in the big bucks. "It was rewarding, but it wasn't a windfall," he says. "It was a way for me to make a living while doing something else, like if I had a part-time job for instance. The subjects are property, and not very valuable property either."[66]

Headaches and sleepiness were common reactions from the studies in which Helms was a subject. The most damage he says he suffered was when he fell asleep and plopped face first into the bleu cheese dressing on a salad he was eating. Not having to endure trauma firsthand has never dampened Helms's desire to advocate for better protection for guinea pigs.

"More than 30 percent of all drugs are found to be too toxic to use in humans," Helms says. "That means people (in Phase I trials) get sick. That doesn't mean they are lied to or intentionally hurt. But, it does mean a lot more people are hurt than we hear about."[67]

Because he believes so many guinea pigs are being hurt. Helms pushes for them to be better protected. For instance, because they are motivated by completely different goals, Helms believes there should be a separate consent process and forms to differentiate subjects who volunteer for a trial because they are sick or altruistic from those who sign up for the money. Helms also thinks, like Dr. Abbott's subjects, that guinea pigs should organize as a profession to secure better conditions, benefits, and wages.

In his quest to stir up the guinea pig fold and encourage them to organize, Helms has run afoul of some deep-pocketed companies. In 1997 Helms and *Harper's* magazine faced a libel suit for a story Helms wrote for *Guinea Pig Zero*, parts of which were reprinted by *Harper's*. Using his magazine to keep guinea pigs up to date on what was happening in their "profession," Helms wrote a report card ranking clinical trials sites so guinea pigs could know which were good places to sign up for studies and at which places a guinea pig was more likely to have an uncomfortable experience or, worse, risk their lives.[68]

The MCP Hahnemann School of Medicine got a very bad report card from Helms. "This unit's problems overwhelm us in their number," Helms wrote in *Guinea Pig Zero*.[69]

While no one took issue with Helms's comments when they were published in *Guinea Pig Zero* with its circulation of about a thousand, when the same comments were sent to the two hundred thousand subscribers of *Harper's*, the MCP Hahnemann School of Medicine hired a lawyer. The attorney told the editors of *Harper's* that because of the false, defamatory, and malicious comments made about the hospital by Helms, he wanted the magazine withdrawn from newsstands, he wanted a retraction, and he wanted an apology. *Harper's* instead ran a clarification that new information about the hospital's consent process was not included in the original article. Helms and *Harper's* were also named in a libel suit, which *Harper's* eventually settled out of court.[70]

The media attention from the lawsuit suited Helms just fine because it helped get people who regulate clinical trials to focus their attention on guinea pigs. The head of what at the time was called the federal Office for Protection from Research Risk, Gary Ellis, said he was an early subscriber to *Guinea Pig Zero* and found that it offered him an "interesting perspective" on research studies and the subjects who take part in them.[71]

Despite the fact that guinea pigs are instrumental in developing lifesaving treatments and drugs, they receive little or no notice from the government or members of the public. Some say that signing up for clinical trials for money is a culture that will probably always operate on the fringes of society. After all most guinea pigs already live on the fringes of American culture: the destitute, the uneducated, the addicted, the desperate. Efforts to improve conditions for guinea pigs, even Helms admits, haven't amounted to much and more than likely won't ever bring about substantive change.

"There have been a few shutdowns of research operations," Helms says. "But that's just political theater."[72]

Others, such as Clough, say that clinical trials for guinea-piggers are safer than they ever have been and probably as safe as they're going to get. But the question of how safe that actually is remains unanswered.

"The clinical trials business model has developed where you have all these companies conducting clinical trials and paying these people to be human subjects," says one lawyer who represents subjects. "So, instead of prisoners, instead of orphans, instead of the mentally retarded, now we're using the poor. How have things improved?"[73]

Chapter 6

GOING GLOBAL

IF YOU'RE LOOKING to conduct a clinical trial in Texas, then the clinical research organization dgdresearch has a pitch for you. On its Web site the San Antonio–based company that specializes in studying diabetes treatments boasts that it opened a new facility on the "city's West side to reach a distinct patient population who are either drug naive or cannot afford medication."[1]

The term "drug naive" is not as bad as it sounds. It's a newly coined term in the pharmacology industry that describes a subject who has not been extensively experimented upon or has not taken a lot of medications in their lifetime.[2] Such subjects are desirable for clinical trials because there are fewer chances that something might interfere with the action of the medication being tested.

Being located near a drug naive population in the United States is a definite business advantage for a CRO conducting a clinical trial. The drug naive are preferred subjects because they help produce more accurate data. Because people in the United States are taking more pharmaceuticals than ever before, there aren't many CROs who can claim the same advantage as dgdresearch. To find large numbers of subjects who are drug naive, as well as to save money and get trials finished faster, pharmaceutical companies and academic research institutions are going global. According to Dr. David Lepay, senior advisor for clinical science at the FDA, "There is no question clinical research is globalizing. It does indeed expedite the product-development process in the United States; that's a positive public health benefit."[3]

Kathy Mayle doesn't think it's such a positive health benefit. A nurse for thirty years, Mayle is the director of the Center for Health Care Diversity at Duquesne University. She has a master's degree in nursing and an MBA from the University of Pittsburgh. Until two years ago she was completely ignorant of how clinical trials were conducted in the third world. But after being on the ground to help with trials and education programs in Nigeria, Nicaragua, and Uganda, she's learned a few things. "They're illiterate, they're not educated, and we don't understand if they're really understanding us," Mayle says about subjects she spent hours explaining consent forms to for a clinical trial in one developing country. "The people were just so happy to get something that was hopeful, just to see someone they thought was a doctor. So they signed the consent. And I'm like, 'These people are hungry. They don't have anything. There are no jobs. I mean we're out in the middle of nowhere. What is going on here?' "[4]

What's going on is that clinical trials are shifting from the United States to the developing world in very high numbers, stoking a fierce debate among medical professionals. Some say offshoring medical testing is a step forward in providing better access to health care to people throughout the world. Others insist that shipping clinical trials overseas exploits and kills vulnerable people in poor countries so that drugs and new medical treatments can be developed for the benefit of rich people living in industrialized nations.

In 1996 86 percent of clinical trials were conducted in the United States. Ten years later that number was down to 57 percent.[5] Judging from the substantial investments large pharmaceutical companies from around the developed world are making to set up shop and test overseas, the trend suggests that clinical trials are likely to find permanent homes in underdeveloped countries. GlaxoSmithKline and AstraZeneca, in England, along with Roche and Novartis, both in Switzerland, are investing $100 million in research in China. Lagging behind but not to be outdone, and with almost $30 billion in drug patents set to expire by 2009 and an additional $160 billion worth of drug patents that will expire by 2015, U.S. companies are also making the move. Eli Lilly, headquartered in Indiana, will spend $300 million in five years in China.[6]

Locating drug naive patients is not the top reason so much investment and clinical trials activity is moving into underdeveloped countries. Just like textile and auto parts manufacturers, IT customer support companies, and makers of everything from Samsonite luggage to Nike running shoes have known for years, it's much cheaper to do business outside the United States and outside developed countries than it is to do business in underdeveloped, or third world countries. Compared to what it costs in money and time in the United States and western Europe, conducting trials in India, Uganda, Brazil, Russia, China, and scores of poor countries is a bargain that can save companies anywhere from 30 to 65 percent on the cost of clinical trials.[7]

On average it costs $6,522 to have a subject go through a clinical trial in the United States. In India for instance, it costs up to 60 percent less per subject.[8] Some savings are generated because facilities and labor are cheaper than they are in the United States.[9] But per-subject cost is not where the real savings come from in clinical trials.

There are no economic reports accurately measuring the impact of government regulations on the cost of a clinical trial. The longer it takes to run a trial the more it costs the sponsor of the trial. That's because of the normal costs to keep a trial going and because of the profits that are lost each day a drug or treatment is in trial and not sold to consumers. Strict FDA regulations for clinical trials in the United States make trials go on longer than if those regulations did not have to be adhered to. For sponsors of clinical trials in countries outside the United States, the FDA will accept data if the trials meet the regulations set forth in the Helsinki Declaration (the 1989 version, not as it was amended in 2000; the Helsinki Declaration is a set of ethical guidelines originally adopted in 1964 to guide doctors in providing treatment in clinical trials and in practice) or regulations established by the host country, whichever are stricter.[10]

According to the U.S. Department of Health and Human Services Office of the Inspector General however, "[the] FDA cannot assure the same level of human subject protections in foreign trials as domestic ones."[11] Even if it could, regulations in clinical trials are almost nonexistent in the developing world.[12] Often there are no rules governing clinical trials not because of oversight but on purpose. Many governments are aware that without Western sponsors of clinical trials coming to test in their countries their populations would have no access to lifesaving or life-enhancing drugs. Zambia, the United Republic of Tanzania, and Malawi are among the many countries that don't even have informed consent regulations. In countries such as Nigeria and South Africa, which do require consent and have institutional review boards, corruption nullifies their effectiveness.[13]

One man, Ilian Ivanov, for instance, oversees the regulations governing clinical trials in Bulgaria. He is simultaneously the regulator and recruiter of companies to come and conduct trials in Bulgaria, and he openly aspires to someday being employed by a pharmaceutical company, just like the man who occupied his post before him. Part of his hundred-dollar monthly paycheck goes toward a bottle of whiskey he keeps at the ready for visitors to his office. Ivanov insists he's no pushover for allowing sponsors of clinical trials to cut corners. Two Bulgarian researchers felt his regulatory wrath once when he caught them conducting trials without government permission. He slapped them with a ten-dollar fine.[14]

Sponsors also save money because it's much easier and cheaper to recruit and retain subjects in other countries than it is in the United States. With recruiting comprising a significant share of the investment in clinical trials in the United States, that money quickly adds up. In a list of the most important factors a company considers when deciding whether or not to move their clinical trials operations overseas, patient availability ranked number one.[15] ("Relevant expertise" of professionals conducting the trials tied for last.[16]) In the United States, sponsors of clinical trials have to run ads and pay doctors to help recruit patients. In Russia patients are recruited into trials by word of mouth.[17] It's so easy because, according to an American working for a company conducting trials in Russia, people in Russia are *eager* to become subjects. It's one of the only ways to gain access to medications that are not subsidized by government programs and that they can't afford.[18] Not only are they lining up to be subjects, the Russians who go into trials are better subjects than their American counterparts. To keep getting Western medications subjects will faithfully show up for appointments, keep diaries if they are required, and comply with most other requests of the study team, no matter how strenuous.[19]

Mayle has seen people in underdeveloped countries wait on line for hours to be part of a trial. She says they're so compliant not merely because they think they'll get a rarely available pill. "It's the fact that, here you are, in the white coat," she says. "You're white, you're American, and there's hope. There's some kind of hope that somebody might help. All they know is there's something wrong with them and they're thinking that they're going to get something, even if it's time, or attention, that sort of thing."[20]

One group that is seemingly even more agreeable and pliable than the subjects in clinical trials is the doctors who recruit subjects on behalf of foreign companies. Some do it because their clinics can obtain badly needed equipment and medication from sponsors of clinical trials, perks that they otherwise would not be able to afford. One clinic in Russia, in order to monitor subjects during a trial, was provided with treadmills by a pharmaceutical company, and they were treasured as a valuable incentive. Sponsors of clinical trials offer cash and trips to doctors who aggressively recruit patients or who sign on as clinical trials investigators. Gift giving is a very effective tool because doctors in developing countries, who often provide the same or better levels of care as Western doctors, are poorly paid by Western standards, usually a few hundred dollars a month. Some foreign doctors are so eager to get aboard the clinical trials gravy train they will work as study monitors, a position traditionally filled by nurses in the United States.[21]

Pharmaceutical companies also offer foreign doctors junkets to Hawaii and other exotic resort destinations if they recruit particularly high numbers of subjects. Such tactics have suddenly turned a lot of foreign physicians into "researchers" who are willing to recruit and treat almost anyone in a clinical trials setting, whether the subject stands to benefit or not. While the money paid by trial sponsors is often publicly earmarked to go into the operating budgets of hospitals and clinics to pay for improvements to patient care, much of it actually ends up being deposited into doctors' personal bank accounts.[22] In Russia, doctors can earn up to ten times their salary conducting clinical trials.[23]

S. P. Kalantri, M.D., is well versed in the challenges doctors and patients must address when a poor hospital in a poor country undertakes a clinical trial for a wealthy foreign drug company. At the hospital in Sevagram, a town in central India famous as a place where Gandhi once lived and as a home to thousands of poisonous vipers, Dr. Kalantri heads up a clinical trial testing a drug from the German drug company Boehringer Ingelheim designed to prevent second strokes. The facility, though considered good by

Indian standards, often suffers power failures and makes do with substandard and old equipment. It's not as bad as other hospitals in the region though, where patients sometimes sleep on mattresses placed on the floor.

Dr. Kalantri views the drug being dispensed in the trial as helpful to his patients given that most of them can't afford any medication at all. Free unproven pills are better than no pills at all for patients trapped in grinding poverty, he reasons. Still, Dr. Kalantri is torn between whether he is acting more as a researcher or a physician as he tries to provide treatment for patients. He's recruited almost one quarter of the total number of patients who have come into the hospital in fifteen months to take part in the trial. He worries, however, that the patients he talks to are too eager to enroll. Most of them, he says, ask *him* if they should enroll rather than deliberating and deciding for themselves. When he informs one potential subject that the drug she would test might not even work she can't grasp the concept. "All drugs work!" she says.[24]

Ethical issues are causing Dr. Kalantri to become selective about saying yes to the companies who call an average of once a week to have a trial conducted at the rural hospital. In turning down some trials because he feels they don't make sense for the population he serves, Dr. Kalantri has earned the scorn of his colleagues, who want the money to pay for improvements to the hospital. He has turned down some trials because they didn't pay enough to cover the costs of lab tests or compensate doctors for the extra time the trials would take. He has turned down others when the amount of money offered was so high it could only be construed as a bribe. Dr. Kalantri considers it important to the integrity of the hospital that he accept payments that correctly compensate only for the services being provided in the trial—a standard not shared by all the hospitals and doctors in the developing world conducting business with the sponsors of clinical trials. When Dr. Kalantri mentions to a representative from Boehringer Ingelheim that the per-patient amount they were paying for the trial seemed high, the company rep told him no one had ever said that before. "Everyone else," he says, "has asked for more."[25]

Hospitals and doctors are not the primary parties in the developing world with their hands out to sponsors of clinical trials. The governments of many developing countries are actively recruiting companies to come and conduct clinical trials. They offer tax breaks and other incentives to companies that will come and run experiments on their populations. India, for instance, makes tax exempt all profits for companies performing in-house research and development, a piece of new legislation that significantly boosts the bottom line of pharmaceutical companies conducting trials. India is more aggressively recruiting Western companies to conduct clinical trials than any other country. Along with generous tax breaks, in January 2006 the country eliminated a law that requires drugs first be tested in the country where they were developed before they can be tested in India. The controversial change eliminates a potential safeguard for India's native population and allows a high number of drug companies to come into the country so they can run trials on India's diverse and vast population of more than one billion people. Or, in the words of one writer, it signals the Indian government's intent to take the lead in the lucrative global clinical trials market and make the county "guinea pig to the world."[26]

To track the studies moving into the country India also established a registry for clinical trials in 2007. Administered through the Indian Council of Medical Research, the registry is voluntary. "To the best of my knowledge," says Sandhya Srinivasan, a medical journalist and editor of the *Indian Journal of Medical Ethics,* "there has not been a significant improvement in the monitoring process."[27]

There are many other regions and countries eager to supplant

India as clinical trials provider to the world. Countries are actually ranked in an "attractiveness index" that allows pharmaceutical companies, CROs, and other sponsors to size up which under-developed nation is best suited to host their next clinical trial. The scorecard created by A. T. Kearney, a consulting company dedicated to corporate growth for its clients, offers a cold-eyed look at the criteria sponsors of clinical trials should consider as they decide on where to conduct a clinical trial in the underdeveloped world. Kearney ranks fifteen countries in terms of their attractiveness and their ability to deliver benefits to sponsors of trials. The rankings are based on five areas of attractiveness: availability of patients; cost effectiveness; expertise of medical personnel; regulatory environment; and facilities and infrastructure. The ranking is on a one to ten scale, with the United States (for reasons of theoretical comparison) scoring better than any country with a 6.8 and Ireland taking last place with 3.86.[28]

Coming in at number three, with a score of 5.55, is Russia. The country offers low costs, a favorable pool of drug naive patients that makes recruitment up to ten times faster than in the United States, and a practice of housing and treating patients with similar symptoms in the same wards for added logistical convenience. The downsides include a high degree of government regulation, a tax on clinical trials, weak intellectual property protection, and potential problems with ethics because the very low doctors' salaries make it likely they might not properly inform patients of potential risks in trials.[29]

India just edges out Russia in grabbing the number two spot with a score of 5.58. The country offers a huge population, expert scientists and doctors who adhere to international treatment standards and whose work is regularly published in international peer-reviewed journals, incentives such as tax exemptions, strong economic growth, and English as the primary language in the country. On the minus side, India, like Russia, doesn't do a great job of protecting intellectual property, the country doesn't allow Phase I clinical trials on healthy patients (although that is likely to change soon), and government regulations requiring that drug companies work with local doctors and hospitals to perform toxicology tests on subjects between testing phases is just one example of the kind of bureaucratic headaches that can cause delays.[30]

The overseas, underdeveloped country that ranks number one as the best choice of any company conducting a clinical trial outside the United States, with a score of 6.10, is China. It offers the biggest urban population on Earth, an enormous overall subject population, and an accompanying large number of existing medical facilities. It also offers almost 1.4 million doctors and more than a million technicians and nurses who are not only well trained, but who also are paid such low salaries that the cost of conducting a trial is cut almost in half. The government is eager to cooperate with Western companies. They have instituted regulations making it easier to run trials and are opening centers to train investigators and support staff. Drawbacks include having to negotiate a confusing government bureaucracy that has requirements like having to obtain a license for every shipment of drugs entering the country rather than a single license for each type of drug. Plus, the country's infrastructure is poor and cultural differences, as well as language problems that cause trials data to be recorded in Chinese rather than English, slow the process down and cost companies money.[31]

One area of consideration not included in the attractiveness index is the impact on the population of the country supplying the subjects. Often, the impact is in the eye of the beholder. In Nigeria the U.S. pharmaceutical company Pfizer is battling an $8.5 billion civil lawsuit and various criminal charges against corporate executives alleging that the company killed eleven children when it ran a 1996 clinical trial for Trovan, an oral meningitis medication, without first getting proper consent from the subjects' families or securing permission from the Nigerian government to test the drug.[32] Pfizer says that, far from using the children as guinea pigs, the company acted heroically and saved the lives of two hundred children during a meningitis outbreak by coming in and dispensing Trovan.

The suit is significant because, although abuses of clinical trials' subjects in poor countries have often been anecdotally claimed, it's perhaps the first time a developing country has brought criminal charges against company executives and researchers for allegedly harming subjects in a clinical trial.[33] (The civil and criminal cases are being tried in Nigeria after a U.S. judge ruled the suit could not be brought before a U.S. court.)

The alleged actions of Pfizer during the meningitis outbreak caused intense outrage in Kano, a predominantly Muslim state in Nigeria, where the testing took place. The deaths helped contribute to parents in several Nigerian states refusing to allow their children to receive polio vaccinations in one of the few areas of the world where the disease is still unchecked.[34] A panel of medical experts appointed by the health minister of Nigeria investigated the incident and wrote a report accusing Pfizer of violating international law when they gave children Trovan. The FDA had approved the drug in 1997 but never approved its use for children. Two years after that approval, the FDA restricted its use even for adults after clinical trials revealed the drug was related to liver damage and even deaths. Trovan was never approved for adults or children in Europe.

For reasons that are still not clear, the incident report by the Nigerian panel of experts regarding the 1996 clinical trial was released a decade after it was written and only after an exhaustive investigation by the *Washington Post* made it public. Also, news reports said that Pfizer allegedly removed all the medical records about the trial from Nigeria. Those actions may have fueled the anger of Nigerian authorities and convinced them to file criminal charges in addition to a civil suit. The language in the lawsuit is strong and extremely accusatory; according to the criminal charges, Pfizer "agreed to do an illegal act," and was "so rash and negligent as to endanger human life."[35]

The lawsuit could signal that U.S. drug companies are wearing out their welcome testing drugs in underdeveloped countries. Nigeria's attorney general, Aliyu Umar, who filed the lawsuit against Pfizer, says, "We realize we are the Third World and we need assistance. But we frown on people who think they can take advantage of us, especially if it's for profit. That's why we decided we needed to take action against Pfizer."[36]

Ben Faneye, M.D., a Nigerian doctor who studied bioethics in the United States and who is a faculty member of the West African Bioethics Training program, says, "For me, I'm not that surprised. I'm coming back from the United States after thirteen years and I'm in that frame of mind where ethics are enforced. To me, I think maybe we're not going far enough."[37]

Dr. Faneye says that while the Nigerian meningitis trials have received a great deal of attention in medical journals and the media in the United States and Europe, on a street level in Nigeria, outside of Kano the case is not widely known. He ascribes that to poor communication in Nigeria and to the national government trying to "put a lid on it" because stirring up populist resentment against Western companies looking to conduct trials in the country is bad for business. Such companies, he says, not only dispense bribes liberally, they also provide badly needed medical treatment in an impoverished country that can barely afford to give people basic care.[38]

Nigeria is one in a long list of countries that appear to be serving as sweatshops for testing Western drugs and procedures, and the Pfizer meningitis story is only one of many such incidents where ethics and rules were allegedly ignored. In India in 2001 a researcher from a prestigious United States university conducted a clinical trial by injecting an experimental cancer drug called M4N into subjects. It was later learned that not only had M4N not been fully tested on animals, but that the subjects had no clue they were even taking part in a clinical trial.[39] A doctor who revealed the testing says he couldn't find an example of such a thing happening anywhere else except perhaps "in concentration camps."[40]

Even if the researcher had gone through the trouble of having subjects sign consent forms, there are some who insist that in the largely illiterate developing world, truly informed consent is impossible. A physician at a hospital in Mumbai, Shashank Joshi, M.D., says informed consent from subjects in India is "a myth according to me . . . Most of the patients sign on the dotted line without understanding the nature and the consequences of what is being administered to them."[41]

Another doctor in India says 90 percent of the time during the consent process people just look at the doctor and ask him or her if they should take part in the trial.[42] A clinical trial for a hepatitis E drug conducted in 2000 in the town of Lalitpur, in Nepal, by the United States Armed Forces Research Institute of Medical Sciences raised serious questions about exactly what consent means in the third world. The drug, licensed by pharmacy giant GlaxoSmithKline, was originally set to be tested on three thousand volunteers in the small town until the local government demanded certain conditions, such as continued access to the drug for subjects after the conclusion of the trial, in order to allow the trial to go forward. The deputy mayor of the town wanted a hospital built after he was told profit sharing of the drug was not an option. But the deal breaker that sent Glaxo packing was negative media attention that strongly suggested a Western drug company had come to town to exploit people. Instead of having to negotiate these demands and deal with growing hostility, the trial was moved so that it could be tested on members of the Royal

Nepalese Army, a group of subjects who wouldn't object to the testing or demand anything in return for being subjects. Not only did recruits have a 44 percent literacy rate,[43] they also were poorly paid members of a totalitarian organization and were completely controlled by military authorities.[44]

When the U.S. National Bioethics Advisory Commission (NBAC) interviewed researchers about consent in developing countries, 13 percent said they didn't think the people they tested in trials were even aware they were part of a study. Asked in the same NBAC review about consent in developing countries, one clinical investigator who was interviewed said flatly: "Informed consent is a joke."[45] After a clinical trial testing HIV transmission in South Africa, 90 percent of the subjects said they felt "forced" to take part in the trial.[46]

In 1995 a study was published that signaled a breakthrough in significantly decreasing the transmission of HIV from pregnant women to their children, but the circumstances of a subsequent study conducted in developing countries raised serious ethical questions. The 1995 study tested a regime of administering an anti-HIV AZT drug called zidovudine to see if it cut transmission of HIV to infants born to infected mothers. The study was carried out in the United States and several other countries. The method included giving the drug orally for months to women before they delivered their children, then administering the drug intravenously during labor, and finally giving the drug to children after they were born. The regime of administering zidovudine cut HIV transmission in one of seven infants, and in newborns by 50 percent in the United States alone. In developing countries, where more than 6 million pregnant women were infected with HIV, the effective, three-step method for administering zidovudine was too expensive to be used widely. In 1997, with funding and support from the U.S. Centers for Disease Control and Prevention along with the National Institutes of Health, researchers set about designing clinical trials that aimed to develop less expensive ways of preventing the transmission of HIV to children in developing countries. The trials tested an abbreviated and cheaper regime of using zidovudine as well as other methods thought to reduce the transmission of HIV, including vitamin A and its extracts, and vaginal washing. The clinical trials involving seventeen thousand women were not conducted the same way in developed countries, such as the United States, as they were in developing countries, however. Subjects in poor countries were not given access to certain drugs during the trial while people in the United States were, and that difference literally meant life and death to children in poor countries whose mothers had HIV.[47]

In the two clinical trials in the United States, HIV-positive women had access to zidovudine, which was proven to be effective. In fifteen out of the sixteen trials in Uganda, Tanzania, Kenya, Thailand, South Africa, and six other impoverished countries, zidovudine was withheld from subjects during the trial and they were given a placebo, which amounts to no treatment at all.[48] This happened even though the company that produced zidovudine offered to donate the drug for free to researchers to use as a comparison drug in the trials.[49] (If a treatment exists it is often used in trials instead of a placebo. Called a "comparison drug," the existing drug is compared to the new drug being tested.)

In April 1997 Peter Lurie, M.D., M.P.H., and Sidney Wolfe, M.D., both with the consumer advocacy organization Public Citizen, held a news conference to call attention to what they called a double standard at work in the trial. A few months later they published an article in the *New England Journal of Medicine* that strongly questioned the ethics of using a placebo and withholding standard, lifesaving treatment in a study involving terminal subjects. The authors maintained that the practice violated the World Medical Association's Helsinki Declaration.

The reaction to the article was a torrent of papers and articles exposing deep divisions in the medical community about what exactly is considered ethical when clinical trials are conducted in developing countries. "There was definitely more attention paid to the lack of an ethical infrastructure for conducting clinical trials in developing countries," Dr. Lurie says, highlighting what he viewed as a positive result of the article.[50]

Along with the attention came considerable dissent in the scientific community. Researchers who designed the trials to find a cheaper alternative to the zidovudine regime insisted their use of a placebo was ethical, and they offered many arguments. One was that using a placebo rather than an active control drug that already exists provides quicker results and that was a crucial consideration in trials where saving time was a priority in addressing a worldwide crisis.

The other argument was more complex and controversial. Researchers defended the practice of using a placebo instead of the existing zidovudine regime because, they said, people in poorer countries would not have had access to the lifesaving regime anyway. NIH's Harold Varmus, M.D., and CDC's David Satcher, M.D., defended the practice by saying, "the assignment to a placebo group does not carry a risk beyond that associated with standard practice."[51]

Lurie, Wolfe, and many others said that rationale was very similar to the rationale used to justify the Tuskegee syphilis clinical trials where black men in Alabama were not treated with penicillin when it became available during the course of the study. Given that Tuskegee is the nadir of moral rectitude in conducting trials in the United States, the comparison is a powerful one. But even on that point there was disagreement.

Doctors said the comparison to Tuskegee was invoked too blithely; using placebos in developing countries, some argued, is not in the same ballpark as Tuskegee. Unlike in the zidovudine study, Tuskegee investigators tricked the subjects so they couldn't even choose whether or not they wanted to be subjects; it targeted vulnerable people in order to recruit and keep them in the study; and it deprived the subjects of medical care in order to achieve the study's goals.[52] The zidovudine trials, some researchers say, do not drop to those same low standards.

Lurie offers a more immediate comparison than Tuskegee. "The same argument [that subjects in poor countries would not have received existing drugs for study comparison] can be made to do placebo studies on people in the United States who don't have insurance. After all, existing treatments are not available to them," he says. "But no one is about to be doing a placebo controlled study on islet cell transplants in the United States because no one would stand for it."[53]

The divisive discourse over whether or not to use placebos in clinical trials in the developing world was supposed to be settled in October 2000. That was when a revision of the Helsinki Declaration would be drafted to clearly define what was and what was not ethical. It was time, Lurie says, to "round up the usual bioethicists" and set new guidelines.[54]

"There are three ways to look at it," Lurie says about revising the declaration. "Helsinki was violated, Helsinki was not violated, or Helsinki was violated but it [the practice of using placebos] was still ethical."[55] The revision to Helsinki came down on endorsing the third option, sort of. The revision had to tread lightly because to always disallow placebos if proven treatments existed could mean that if a clinical trial for something innocuous like nasal decongestants, for example, were conducted then the sponsor of the trial would have to compare it to existing nasal decongestants, a potentially complicated and burdensome standard to uphold. Paragraph 20 of the Helsinki Declaration was rewritten to say, "The benefits, risks, burdens and effectiveness of a new method should be tested against those of the best current prophylactic, diagnostic, and therapeutic methods." But a footnote to that clear language was also included. The footnote said two things: First, a placebo was ethical "where for compelling and scientifically sound methodological reasons its use is necessary," which addressed the need for speed in using a placebo in the zidovudine trials. The second part of the footnote put the sponsors of clinical trials for new nasal decongestants at ease. It said a placebo was ethical "where a . . . method is being investigated for a minor condition and the patients who receive a placebo will not be subject to any additional risk of serious or irreversible harm."[56]

When asked what compelled researchers to use a placebo rather than a proven treatment in the zidovudine trials in the first place, Lurie puts forward two theories. Using placebos in the late 1990s, he says, was simply standard practice in clinical trials.

Robert Temple, the director of medical policy at the FDA's Center for Drug Evaluation and Research, has been with the agency for more than thirty years. He is one of the most influential drug regulators in the world, and his preference for how trials should be conducted resonates with anyone designing studies. Temple strongly advocates using placebos in clinical trials.[57] He is quoted as calling the ethics behind the amendment to paragraph 20 of the Helsinki Declaration "bizarre."[58] He disagreed with the new policy and warned it could end development of entire categories of new drugs.

Temple and the FDA went further than merely disagreeing with the revision. The agency issued a paper in March 2001 that reflects the FDA's position to this day. "The FDA has not taken action to incorporate this revision into its regulations," it said regarding guidelines for the pharmaceutical industry. "The action of the World Medical Association [which drafts the declaration] did not change FDA regulations."[59] To be even more blunt about its position, in January 2001 the FDA had an internal meeting the topic of which was: "Use of placebo-controls in life-threatening diseases: Is the developing world the answer?"[60]

In the end the controversy over the zidovudine trials meant using placebos in clinical trials in the developing world was shaken but not knocked off as the preference of most researchers. In trials conducted in the United States and the developed world, however, using placebos was already fading out as a preferred research method in trials for treatments of life-threatening conditions when a standard treatment existed.

In recent years some of the only known instances of placebos being used in trials in the United States where subjects were at high risk involved studying methadone and its effect upon the success rate in drug withdrawal treatment, and a study that compared the use of sterile needles to used syringes in significantly stemming the spread of diseases such as hepatitis C among drug addicts. But those trials are hardly representative of how often placebos are used in U.S. trials testing blockbuster drugs intended for mainstream consumption because they were conducted on marginalized, "disempowered" drug addicts.[61]

Lurie dismisses any evil intent on behalf of the researchers involved in the zidovudine trials to make a profit. He prefers to think the researchers had good intentions, even if they employed questionable practices. "This wasn't a trial for a drug company," he says. "This was the NIH and the CDC. The trials were done by not-for-profit types and academicians. It wasn't about money."[62]

Another case study demonstrates that when trials in the developing world are about money, evil intent appears to creep more definitively into the equation.

In 2001 the FDA was considering whether to approve an application from a Pennsylvania biotechnology company to test a drug on infants in Latin America that would treat a potentially fatal lung condition. The company, Discovery Labs, was asking to give some of the potential subjects in the clinical trial a placebo, or no treatment at all even though existing drugs could be tested for comparison and would keep children from dying of the lung condition.

The president of Discovery, Robert Capetola, said using a placebo in one-third of the trials could cut eighteen months off how long it took to complete the studies. "We think it would be totally un-ethical not to conclude it and get it to patients quicker," he said about the trial.[63]

Another rationale that Capetola offered was that using a placebo would not leave children any worse off than they already were be-cause children didn't receive any treatment at all in most Latin American hospitals. In fact, Capetola said, the infants in the study would get better care than without the trial because Discovery would donate antibiotics and ventilators to trial sites.[64] However, by contrast, all infants in the trial sites slated for Europe would re-ceive existing, approved treatments to test against the new drug.

Even though Temple and the FDA still favored placebo trials for their expedience and accuracy, Discovery faced a tough battle within the agency to win permission for a placebo trial in a devel-oping country so soon after the controversy over the HIV/zi-dovudine trials. An internal FDA document about Discovery's application was unambiguous in saying that to give a placebo to children who might die without treatment is "considered uneth-ical in the USA." It was also unethical in the rest of the world, according to the recent amendment to Helsinki Declaration that was not recognized, but apparently not wholly refuted, by the FDA.

Consumer advocacy groups, including Public Citizen, lashed out against the idea of another placebo trial that could endanger or even end the lives of sick infants. The hue and cry was heard loud and clear. In April 2001 the FDA denied Discovery's appli-cation without comment.[65] Discovery decided to redesign the study so that all subjects received active control medications for comparison to the new medication. The change was hailed as a rare success in trying to achieve a single accepted standard for using placebos in trials no matter where they took place. "This should make it clear to all clinical researchers that developing countries are not to be used as a dumping ground for unethical research," said a news release from Public Citizen Health Research Group after the trial design change was announced. "There should be no question now that exploiting the poverty of developing country residents is completely unacceptable. We hope that no company will be so foolhardy as to consider such exploitative research again."[66]

With financial forces acting so powerfully to drive increasing medical research in poor countries, the question turns from how to stop "exploitative" research to how to better manage it so that it's not so harmful to subjects. Clinical trials are a bonanza of cash and/or equipment and medications for governments, hospitals, and researchers in poor, developing countries and a way to generate profits by cutting the costs of trials for CROs and pharmaceutical and medical device companies in the developed world. But what about the subjects? What, if anything, are the subjects who are putting their health and lives on the line getting out of the deal?

Subjects in developing countries receive medical care from doctors that they otherwise would probably not have access to. They receive treatment, at least for a little while, with a drug or therapy (even if they are experimental) that they otherwise could never get. Those are benefits by happenstance, however.

There are no set standards and there is little agreement among researchers, government agencies, and companies on guaranteeing continued care for subjects after a trial is concluded. In the United States and other Western countries it's common practice for the sponsors of trials to continue dispensing drugs or treatment after the trial is completed and before the drug or treatment is made available to the general public. Once it's made available, subjects can get their hands on the drug or treatment through their doctor or pay for it with insurance. In the developing world, the decision whether participants will be provided access to medications, or anything more, is made by the sponsor of a trial once their participation comes to an end. Even then, if a drug or treatment is provided to bridge the gap until it's made available, in developing countries it's just a temporary measure. A company is not required to sell its discovery in the country in which it was tested. Even if they do make it available, in many developing countries former subjects usually can't afford to buy it. The practice is called "parachute research," when a company drops into a country, conducts its trials, then leaves without a trace.[67]

"The whole AIDS thing and the reason why I'm so upset is that once you start the drugs for AIDS then you have to take them for the rest of your life," Mayle says. "If you stop it, what happens is that the virus can morph into something that the industry standard [drug or treatment] will not ever correct to help you. So what's happening is they get all these people in a third world country, they give them some treatment, then after the research is done the researcher doesn't feel a responsibility to continue the drug and the person can't afford it. So [the subject] is stuck with no way of continuing their medication. It's horrible. It's horrible that these people's lives are dispensable. I get very upset."[68]

Pharmaceutical giant Merck has pockets deep enough to fund a special program that makes life-enhancing drugs available to needy people in countries where they test and where the drug they tested is not sold. But Louis Lange, M.D.—the head of a small biotech company, CV Therapeutics, that developed a new drug for angina and tested it on poor subjects in Eastern Europe and Russia—doesn't have the resources of Merck. He's not sure what to do for the subjects in the trial that helped him develop his drug and start his company on the road to success but he says, "We are concerned."[69] While Lange is conflicted about not being able to supply drugs to the impoverished people he is running tests on, he rightly points out that he's running a business and not a charity. "People who run corporations," says Robert Hinkley, an expert in business ethics, "have a legal duty to shareholders, and that duty is to make money. Failing this duty can leave directors and officers open to being sued by shareholders."[70] In other words, the business of business is, by law, to make money.

Lange is not alone in struggling with the ethical quandary of caring for subjects after trials are finished. "Do we have an obligation to everyone in the trial or to everyone in the community, the province, the nation, the region of the world?" asks Ruth Faden, Ph.D., a bioethicist at Johns Hopkins University. "We haven't really figured this out."[71]

For many the issue of whether companies have more of a responsibility for meeting the commercial demands of clinical research over providing humane treatment to those who contribute directly to that research is unresolved. "Many physician investigators feel uncomfortable with the idea of using patients in studies then not being able to continue to help them when the trial ends," Dr. Faden says. "We seem to have hit a wall of moral unease. In the end, I'm not exactly sure where we ought to end up."[72]

Use of placebos and whether to provide continued care for subjects are only two areas of moral unease accompanying the practice of conducting more and more clinical trials in developing countries. Corporations also come under fire, because when they test unproven drugs and treatments on human beings critics are more prone to express their rage over perceived exploitation than if a business is, say, making widgets and paying foreign workers a low wage. The damage inflicted in the clinical trials business seems more immediate and personal. To tamp down this criticism many large pharmaceutical companies, such as Merck, Pfizer, Johnson & Johnson, and others, earmark part of the profits they make from doing business in underdeveloped countries to support hospitals, clinics, schools, training, and additional humanitarian aid.

Critics contend that even though such giving is directly beneficial to the populations of poor countries, for U.S. and European corporations that kind of spending is part of the cost of generating goodwill in a foreign country where they wish to set up shop or of maintaining a good image in an industry where mistakes can generate extremely negative media attention.

Some experts take a more pragmatic stance on who bears responsibility for what happens in clinical trials in underdeveloped countries. In the opinion of Ezekiel J. Emanuel, M.D., corporations are not the only ones at fault. "They [subjects] have an obligation to protect their own self-interest," he says about supposed lapses in the informed consent process. "If you rent a car, do you read all the paperwork they give you? Most people don't read all the information on a car rental agreement. The information is there; they have access to it. I find the histrionics surrounding [human] research tiring. Once it's the body it becomes different than anything else."[73]

"The main business of clinical research is not enhancing or saving lives but acquiring stuff: data," says journalist Sonia Shah in her influential book *The Body Hunters*, in which she writes critically of big drug companies. "It is an industry, not a social service. The people who sponsor and direct clinical trials do it for the data, not to please patients or help bolster ailing health facilities, although they may point to these side effects to justify their activities. Their motives don't make them corrupt or mercenary, either, just regular, self-protective humans like the rest of us."[74]

Others, such as Kathy Mayle, point to the front line of clinical trials and say researchers should ensure that subjects in developing countries are treated as fairly as their counterparts in developed countries. Mayle says the lack of infrastructure in poor countries puts the onus squarely on researchers to conduct trials ethically and protect the interest of subjects. But, similar to corporations, researchers in clinical trials are not one-on-one medical caregivers. "Research being done in developing countries . . . is not really for the benefit of those people [the subjects]," bioethicist Solomon Benatar told Sonia Shah. "It may happen to be, for the few people lucky enough to get into the trial. But the reason the researcher is coming to that country is more often than not because somebody is willing to pay for the study. Somebody wants an answer to a question. The data is valuable either academically or commercially."[75]

For researchers working in underdeveloped countries, turning away sponsors of clinical trials for ethical lapses could prove devastating to their efforts to provide even basic care in substandard hospitals and clinics. Plus, the experimental "treatment" being delivered during the trial is a valuable resource. "These universities and hospitals are really strapped for cash," Peter Lurie says. "If a company comes in with $2 million in hard currency for a clinical trial, it's hard to say no. If they say yes, half the people will get a drug that might work compared to no one getting any treatment at all. It's hard to say no."[76]

Countries that put out the welcome mat to sponsors of clinical trials are also well motivated. The first concern of such governments is to gain medical treatment, investment, scientific expertise, and other desperately needed resources that accompany clinical trials. They could lose these benefits if they were to regulate so strongly against clinical trials that sponsors took their studies—and their largesse—elsewhere. The FDA is too swamped trying to track and regulate the clinical trials conducted in the United States to even try to carefully monitor trials taking place in the rest of the world. If the agency were to take a harder line on regulations overseas it could significantly curtail the development of drugs that not only make money for the companies that develop them, but provide lifesaving and life-enhancing treatment to people suffering in the United States and throughout the world.

Some say the media has been lax in telling the story of how drugs and treatments are tested in poor countries. They argue that if more people in the developed world knew what was taking place they would put pressure on regulators, corporations, researchers, and foreign governments to enforce stricter ethics standards and safeguard subjects in the third world. On December 17, 2000, the *Washington Post* published the first of a six-part series that reported on the unethical treatment of subjects and outright abuses of subjects in clinical trials sponsored by U.S.-based drug companies in the developing world.[77] The series was very effective in raising public awareness.

In 2002 U.S. representative Thomas Lantos, a Democrat from California, mentioned the articles in the text of a bill he sponsored called the "Safe Overseas Human Testing Act." The bill was scrupulous in showing an understanding of the issues that might compromise the safety of subjects enrolled in foreign clinical trials sponsored by U.S. researchers. "International and most foreign-country legal protections do not adequately shield participants in clinical investigations of a new drug or device from unethical, dangerous, or unscrupulous research practices." The bill goes on to say, "Some researchers exploit the fragile regulatory systems, high illiteracy rates, and public health failures of developing countries to test their experimental drugs and devices on misinformed and unwilling human participants." In urging new regulations the bill flatly stated, "While Federal regulation should accelerate, whenever possible, the delivery from laboratory to patients of new drugs which are designed to treat devastating illnesses, existing law permits manufacturers to profit from the misery and pain of uninformed, misinformed, and unwilling patients in developing countries."[78]

The bill sought to prevent U.S. researchers from sending ex-perimental drugs to developing countries for testing unless they first shared the to-date details of the trials with U.S. regulators. To get a license just to ship the drugs out of the United States, the sponsors of a trial would also have to prove that an ethics com-mittee, such as an IRB, had reviewed and approved the design of the study.[79] "It is important that the United States government do all it can to help protect human beings in poor countries who are vulnerable to unethical biomedical and behavioral researchers," Representative Lantos said at the time. "These tests must be con-ducted under standards no less rigorous than if these tests were conducted in the United States."[80]

The bill was added as an amendment to the Export Admin-istration Act that was being considered by the House Commit-tee on International Relations during the 106th Congress. It did not get voted on in the final version of the overall bill. The bill was reintroduced in the 107th Congress. It met the same fate as in the previous session of Congress. The third time was not a charm when the bill came before the 109th Congress, where it again died. As of February 2009 the bill has not been enacted.[81]

The complexities of global clinical trials mirror the complexi-ties of clinical trials as they have been conducted in the United States and throughout the world down through time. There are competing forces vying for information, discovery, money, and fame all in the name of science. Whatever the solution to improv-ing the treatment of subjects in overseas clinical trials, it will have to start—and may even end—with the same thing that will im-prove the treatment of subjects in U.S. clinical trials: information.

"The government means well," says Dr. Faneye about the poor state of clinical trials regulation in Nigeria. "The researchers want to do well. We're talking about the dignity of human subjects, though. You can't always rely on the goodwill of others. The best way to improve things in Nigeria is not a lawsuit. It is through a people's awareness program. Tell people, give them the information, and they will make things improve."[82]

Chapter 7

THE PERFECT LABORATORY
FOR CLINICAL TRIALS

THERE IS MUCH more to Uganda than Idi Amin. It is a
country of 28 million people in sub-Saharan East Africa
whose medical establishment is openly deliberating and wrestling
with the thorny issues and challenges of ethically managing clinical trials in a place that suffers grinding poverty.

Uganda is home to one of the most sophisticated research institutions devoted to clinical trials ever designed, employing some of
the most stringent medical and ethical standards in the world. At
the same time, pharmaceutical companies from the United States
and all over the world run rampant throughout Uganda recruiting
subjects for clinical trials with methods that are sometimes far from
ethical. Doctors at cash-strapped clinics and hospitals say they welcome any company or research institution that brings them a clinical trial, whether they operate ethically or not, because they also
bring technology and drugs to treat people who are literally dying
by the thousands. For these reasons and many more, Uganda is the
perfect laboratory to study clinical trials.

Like many African countries, Uganda has long battled malaria
and tuberculosis. And even though millions of native people died
from these diseases (among others) for centuries, companies and
research institutions did not conduct very many clinical trials in
Uganda addressing these conditions. That's because there's no
profit-generating market for drugs and treatments for malaria

and tuberculosis. Those diseases are not prevalent in the affluent Western world. It's HIV and AIDS, diseases with high rates in the United States and other developed, drug-buying countries, that brought clinical trials to Uganda.

The HIV infection rate among adults in Uganda is 6.3 percent.[1] The disease has killed more than one million people.[2] (Half a million people have died of AIDS in the United States,[3] but it has ten times the population of Uganda.) AIDS has created almost two million orphans in the country.[4] As early as 1995, almost 90 percent of all men and women living in Uganda knew someone infected with HIV.[5] Other countries have higher rates and more sobering numbers of HIV- and AIDS-related deaths. What sets Uganda apart from other countries, and what is attracting the attention and investment of those who conduct clinical trials, is the country's openness about the disease and its aggressive efforts to provide treatment and prevention. Uganda is one of the only countries in the world that, through governmental programs and direct intervention, actually reduced the number of HIV/AIDS cases in the country. They did this, in part, by reducing the social stigma of HIV and AIDS. Through an innovative educational program called ABC (standing for abstinence, be faithful, and condom use), HIV rates were reduced from 15 percent of the population in the early 1990s to about 5 percent in 2001.[6] The overall efforts at HIV/AIDS awareness education in Uganda can be favorably compared to programs in the United States that educate people about the dangers of smoking.[7]

Such success is due in no small measure to the fact that, in myriad and fascinating ways, Uganda defies the clichés of a backwater third world country. It is unique among nations in Africa and throughout the world. The capital city of Kampala, for instance, is home to 2 million people: during each workday that number doubles. There are maybe ten traffic lights, tops, in the entire city, yet there are few accidents even though men on motorbikes scratch

out a living ferrying passengers around, darting in and out of traffic with the skill and instincts of mosquitoes scurrying across the
surface of a pond. The motorcyclists are called *boda-boda*, African
patois for border-border. They got their start as smugglers working
the borders of Kenya in and around Nairobi and the Sudan, bringing whatever could be sold into a country laid waste by Idi Amin
and subsequent dictators who killed more than 4 million Ugandans
in the 1970s and 1980s. Once political stability came to Uganda in
the late 1990s, instead of locking up the *boda-boda*, the government
legalized them so they could work as short-trip taxi drivers, giving
young men a way to earn a few shillings and giving people a way
to get from work to home and back in a country lacking decent
roads and even basic infrastructure. That's how things are done in
Uganda. They find a way, using what they have, to make things
work. They take pride in doing it on their own. Uganda leads
Africa in entrepreneurship.

Despite this ingenuity, this landlocked country where gas is
about $8 a gallon remains very poor. There are entire buildings
throughout Kampala and the countryside painted top to bottom
by companies that use them as billboards. For instance, MTN, the
cell phone company, will paint a building yellow and blue and
put its logo all over it. The owners of the buildings don't license
their surface space to MTN for any money; they do it for the
paint. The average per capita income in Uganda is $330 a year,
less than $1 per day. But that's not an economic death sentence
to people in Uganda. It's a challenge to be creative. If there's a
way to get ahead, they'll find it.

The Ugandan government's dedication to HIV/AIDS treatment
and prevention, and its openness to addressing the disease head-on
despite having few resources, has long made it fertile ground for
clinical trials. Some of those trials, however, were utter failures.

According to a report from the Netherlands-based Centre for
Research on Multinational Corporations, one trial testing the

drug nevirapine to prevent mother-to-child HIV transmission, sponsored by the company Boehringer Ingelheim and the NIH, involved a rash of unethical behavior and was stopped in 2003 after six years. Deviations from ethical standards included: investigators failing to get proper consent from subjects; not reporting issues that put lives at risk and at times killed people; not reporting fourteen fatalities; and researchers failing to disclose literally thousands of cases of adverse reactions to the drug being tested. Boehringer Ingelheim went so far as to ask the NIH to shred a copy of the report about the trial before the FDA could get a look at it. When the litany of violations became public the drug company withdrew its application for approval of the drug.[8]

In 2005, just as the country was starting to embrace clinical research to help address its AIDS epidemic, a trial was halted that resonates throughout the country's medical establishment to this day. A multisite trial funded by a $24 million grant from the Bill and Melinda Gates Foundation and run by a partnership of Eastern Virginia Medical School and the U.S. Agency for International Development (USAID)[9] was begun to study the use of a microbicidal gel to prevent the transmission of HIV to women. More than a thousand subjects were recruited in Uganda, India, South Africa, and other countries. The trial was abruptly halted in January 2007 when results revealed that thirty-five of the women testing the gel became infected with HIV, a higher rate than those receiving a placebo.[10] The cause of the increased HIV infections among the subjects remains unclear but is still being investigated. All the higher infection rates took place at the African sites, not at the sites in India, and that raised the ire of experts speaking to the media about the exploitation of African trials' subjects by Western medical experts.[11]

Months after the trials were stopped and before any conclusions were reached, Ugandan journalist and advocate Moses Paul Sserwanga wrote on his blog that many politicians in Uganda were concerned that people were being used as "guinea pigs for experiments that could not be done in Europe and America." He went on to say, "Uganda doesn't have a legal framework to regulate the conduct of biomedical research . . . Any country wishing to take part in scientific research involving human beings needs to have a national plan to address ethical and sometimes criminal issues because medical research should not be conducted in isolation of fundamental human rights."[12] Those comments earned some rebuke. One blogger identified as Lucio on Sserwanga's Web site wrote, "I find many of your comments inflammatory . . . you paint scientists as racist Nazis. Shame."[13]

Aside from generating vitriolic back and forth, the trial caused the Ugandan medical establishment to give weight and consideration to the ethics of clinical trials conducted in their country. The debate about how to impose and enforce ethical standards in clinical trials is unresolved but, unlike many other developing countries, at least the discussion is taking place.

One medical center sets the high standard by which clinical trials should be conducted not only in Uganda, but anywhere in the world. Thirty miles south of the capital city of Kampala, near Entebbe, the International AIDS Vaccine Initiative (IAVI) is located on a sprawling, multiuse campus overlooking the majesty of Lake Victoria. For more than six years researchers at IAVI, starting in Uganda and now extending to twenty locations around the globe, have been conducting research and clinical trials to find a vaccine for HIV/AIDS.

More than twenty-five fellowship recipients from Pfizer volunteer at IAVI. Given such lofty credentials, it was no accident that IAVI initiated its international efforts to search for an AIDS vaccine in Uganda, according to Pontiano Kaleebu, M.D., Ph.D., a Ugandan who is IAVI's principal investigator. "Uganda has been accepting," he says while seated with a cup of tea in a thatched gazebo on the IAVI grounds, "the AIDS problem has been open.

Countries have been quiet about the problem they have, but not Uganda. The government has been open. The people have been open. We have been welcoming research to see that we can solve the problem we have. We have said we have to be part of solving the problem. We cannot let others do this for us. So that openness in the political environment and in the science environment has all been useful in the decision to come here."[14]

The facilities at Entebbe, housed at the Uganda Virus Research Institute, are among the most advanced in the world. In a country where air conditioning is very rare, they have an IT center with banks of servers kept so chilled that the full-time IT manager has to wear a jacket to stay comfortable while he works. All collected tissue and blood samples are stored using state of the art technology. Immersed in tanks of liquid nitrogen and housed in a separate building, probes measure the temperature of each sample every two minutes. That data is then recorded every thirty minutes to ensure that auditors have clear records of sample viability. Before they got the probes, technicians took the readings by hand.

IAVI personnel conduct in-depth outreach seminars to recruit subjects. They go out to rural villages and town centers, attracting up to three hundred people, providing information and answering any and all questions people have. Then they stay behind and interview people one-on-one after the seminars and invite them to the clinic for a physical screening if they think they will qualify. If they pass the physical, potential subjects are permitted to take the consent form home and study it at their leisure before they sign and agree to take part. The consent forms that the subjects receive, Dr. Kaleebu says, are translated from English into Luganda, the country's indigenous language, then back into English from the Luganda version to make double sure the translation is accurate by independent translators not involved in the success or failure of the trials. In the end, one in five people who go through a second physical screening are eventually recruited to become subjects.

Complementing the rigor involved in the consent process and the forward-looking technology, the thirty-five people employed at IAVI are experts in their chosen fields. They seem not only professionally but also personally dedicated to the work they're doing. Dr. Kaleebu, as an example, received his medical degree from Makerere University Medical School in Kampala as well as a degree in immunology and a Ph.D. at London University. He is the chairman of the African AIDS Vaccine Program, he sits on the boards of the South African AIDS Vaccine Initiative (SAAVI) and the AIDS Vaccine Advocacy Coalition (AVAC) in New York, and he is a Visiting Reader, Imperial College, University of London. The administrator at IAVI is a young man named Peter Ssamula Kiwanuka. Before coming to IAVI he was the human resources director for the auto conglomerate Daimler in Uganda. He was drawn to dedicate himself to vaccine research after four of his siblings died of AIDS.[15]

That firsthand familiarity with the devastation of AIDS is what brings many subjects to IAVI. Because it is conducting a vaccine trial, all of the subjects are healthy individuals who do not have HIV or AIDS. "Generally these are ordinary people," Dr. Kaleebu says about the two hundred subjects who are so far enrolled at IAVI's Entebbe site. "There is no uniqueness about them. They're teachers, they're people working in offices, people working in trade, people working in hospitals, they are students so it's a wide sort of range, a cross-section of people who come."[16]

IAVI has made every effort to secure public endorsement of the trial because previous trials that lacked public support failed. Dr. Kaleebu was an investigator on the 1999 microbicide trial and he says one issue that was never overcome in that study was public suspicion. "People were saying, 'Why are these trials coming here? Why are they being done here? Are we being treated as guinea pigs?'" Dr. Kaleebu recalls. "Those guinea pig stories. They thought this vaccine is going to cause harm. They were asking why isn't it done in the developed countries?"[17]

IAVI's success in everything from stringently adhering to World Health Organization standards to securing positive media coverage of their trial has a downside. They have set the bar for clinical trials very high in Uganda. Other companies or research institutions are not as adequately funded and, lacking the international connections and support of IAVI, can't hope to measure up to the standard IAVI sets. Dr. Kaleebu is aware that the IAVI model might not be the standard on which all other Ugandan clinical trials should be modeled because to do so is simply not practical. "We are all aiming very high," Dr. Kaleebu says. "I think the time will come where we'll say, 'Hmm, do we need all this?' We are not going to compromise on consent. But I think what has come in is this GCP—good clinical practice. In some cases it [calls for] too much paperwork. We have done a few studies that have not followed this highest requirement [of GCP] and have done quite well. So what is the standard? This is a debate we will have as we go ahead."[18]

Some companies and research institutions conducting clinical trials in Uganda are apparently not bothering with the debate about ethical standards. They're just going ahead. Three times in the last two years representatives from pharmaceutical companies have driven up to Charles's house offering him money and favors to test their experimental HIV drugs.[19] Charles lives in Gayaza, a small town of red dirt roads, brick houses, and crumbling shacks on the outskirts of Kampala. A single father since his wife died of AIDS, Charles is raising six children, one of whom has HIV. He was diagnosed with HIV almost three years ago at the age of forty-three. When he got sick, Charles went to Mulago Hospital, a state-funded facility that luckily has a nearby clinic. Once a month he walks five miles to the clinic to get Nevipan, Zerit, and

Lamivudine—donated pills that make up the drug cocktail that keep him and his daughter alive—then walks home.

Charles isn't sure which companies the drug reps who visited him work for. He has no idea how they even found out where he lives. People in Uganda do not have numbers on their houses. Everyone uses a post office box. To locate him would require access to detailed personal information, like the kind found in medical records. Charles only knows the drug reps were from three different companies, they were white, they were American, and they were prepared to be very generous. "They offered me money," Charles says. "They offered to fix my house if I would take their drugs."[20] Charles fires bricks for a living. It is hard, tedious, physically demanding, poorly paying work. His doctor tells him that he's too sick to be doing such work and that it's putting his already fragile health in further jeopardy. Charles has no choice. Without his wages, and a little charitable help that he receives, he and his children would be utterly destitute. Despite the offers of money and help, Charles turned each of the drug companies down cold. "The drugs I am taking are working," he says. "I have no reason to take their drugs."[21] He says however, that he is certain many other people with HIV have agreed to test drugs because the money the drug companies are offering is hard for most people to resist.

Charles is typical of other Ugandans who suffer from HIV and AIDS in at least the way he was recruited to take part in a clinical trial. Jackson is a thirty-year-old native of Kampala who has been enrolled since 1992 in a clinical trial sponsored by a U.S. drug company testing antiretroviral drugs. When he first considered signing up for the trial he was scared of what might happen. But he was led to talk to an investigator about experimental medication because the aspirin he was taking to fend off the HIV symptoms was not working and he had no money for treatment. "I was falling asleep at work and couldn't work after a time," he says in Luganda through an interpreter.[22]

He met once with an investigator for a trial who violated almost every ethical standard of subject recruitment. She told him he could either take the drugs the company was offering or he could die. She told him that he would take the drugs for three months and after that would receive no more care or medication related to the trial and that he would be on his own. Jackson was also told that once he signed a consent form he had to stay enrolled in the trial and on the drugs until it ended. The investigator also ran down a long list of potential side effects. Jackson was intimidated by the possibility of lethargy, vomiting, and headaches. He spoke to his wife, who was also HIV positive and who had already enrolled in the trial. She put her foot down, side effects or no side effects. "It took my wife to convince me,"[23] Jackson says with a laugh. As he was nearing the end of the three months Jackson says the trial was extended. He now gives blood once every three months and is still enrolled.

When Rose, a thirty-three-year-old poultry farmer, started getting dizzy in the sun and losing her strength she knew she was sick. After tests at a hospital revealed HIV, she was referred to an investigator who was conducting a clinical trial. She met with a Ugandan native who was working for an American drug company. He told her she would take experimental medication for eighteen days. She was told she could stop at any time if the drugs made her sick. She agreed to enroll and was given two consent forms, one in Luganda and one in English, a language she barely knew how to speak and couldn't read. She was told the forms were identical but she was given only the English version to sign.

The drugs gave her uncontrollable nausea and made her so tired she could barely get out of bed. Because she was poor, and realizing there was nothing else she could do to treat her HIV, she continued taking the medication. After six months the drugs finally started making her feel better. Considering her a successful subject and wanting to retain her in the study, Rose says the investigator told her that if she dropped out of the trial she would have to pay for the medical care she'd received over the past six months. Rose, who wears a T-shirt from the National Association of Women with HIV with the words "Uganda AIDS Commission" on it, says during the six months she was in the trial she did a little research. "I read about human rights and the rights of medical subjects," she says, "and I told them I knew they could not do that."[24] Rose is now in her sixth year as a subject in the trial.

Besides being severely ill and wanting treatment, Rose says what convinced her the trial would be safe was that the meds being tested were from the United States. "All I knew was that the drugs were from America," Rose says. "Some people make drugs not up to standards. Some drugs from other places do bad things, liver damage. If it's from America, it's good."[25]

Annett is a soft-spoken thirty-seven-year-old who used to work as a cleaver for a butcher. For over four years she's been enrolled in a clinical trial testing a mixture of drugs to treat her HIV. She, like Rose, was asked to sign only the English version of a consent form. Because she's unable to read either English or Luganda, a Ugandan doctor working for the American pharmaceutical company sponsoring the trial signed the consent form for her. She was told by the same doctor, "If you take the drugs, they will work. If you don't take them they will not work."[26] The drugs have made her feel healthy. She says she's grateful to be enrolled because now she can look for a job and, if she gets one, she can keep it because she has the strength to work. The trial, however, had some setbacks. It is ending in March 2009, and Annett is promised she will be referred elsewhere for free or low-cost anti-retroviral medication, although there are no guarantees. Her family disagreed with her decision to enroll in the trial and literally disowned her for it. She thought about it carefully and became a subject anyway. "When they saw that I did not die," Annett says, "they love me again."[27] One day a team of researchers from the study arrived at her place of work in a truck emblazoned with the name of the HIV trial they were conducting.[28] Even though she lost her job as a result, she stayed in the study.

The most startling trait these subjects share is not that they were treated in such an utterly shabby manner by the researchers sponsoring and conducting the trials they are enrolled in. It's that even knowing that their rights as subjects and as people were grossly violated they remain incredibly grateful to be in the trials they are in. The medication is saving their lives. They know it. Annett says she would tell other people with HIV to become subjects in a clinical trial because they might get treatment. Jackson says his only regret about the trial has nothing to do with the violation of his rights. It's that while he didn't suffer any side effects, his wife—the one who convinced him to get over his fear of side effects and enroll—is suffering through severe reactions.

These people, these subjects, are not grateful out of ignorance or naiveté. They know their rights were violated. They also know that being sick with a fatal disease in a country where per capita health-care spending is a little more than five cents per day[29] makes the sanctity of such rights a luxury. But, in stark contrast to the United States, where protecting individual rights is sacrosanct, people in Uganda, like many countries outside the Western world, tend to think more communally than individually. Ugandans will typically refer to cousins they are particularly close to as "brother" or "sister" as a way of extending one's family, of belonging to a larger group, says Father John Mary Mooka (pronounced Moe-ka), a Catholic priest from Uganda who is studying for his Ph.D. in bioethics at Duquesne University in Pittsburgh. To violate the letter of the law governing the rights of a few if doing so benefits many is viewed as an acceptable tradeoff in Uganda.

Desperate and poor subjects looking for health-care options view such bargaining to achieve the best overall results in combating HIV and the nation's other health problems as a viable

option. Many in Uganda's medical establishment would welcome clinical trials into their institutions if it meant improved
treatment for the sick.

As the associate director of the Nsambya Hospital HIV/AIDS
clinic in Kampala, Paul Simon Mayanja is in charge of helping
people in this area of the city receive treatment for HIV/AIDS
and related diseases. When asked, he says he would welcome a
clinical trial to his clinic as a "good Samaritan,"[30] provided the
trial was reputable and ethical.

It's easy to see why. Outside the clinic on a Tuesday morning
more than fifty men, women, and children sit silently and pa-
tiently on benches or on the concrete floor outside the clinic that
was recently built with U.S.-based corporate assistance. Nurses in
old-style, tricornered caps and doctors in white lab coats usher
people into the clinic after grabbing their folders from stacks of
medical records sitting unmonitored and unsecured at the edge
of a covered, outdoor waiting area. Some patients come once a
month for antiretroviral drugs at little or no cost, some are examined and receive blood testing for HIV/AIDS, malaria, and liver
function, while still others receive treatment for tuberculosis and
other AIDS-related illnesses.

A pair of numbers related to the Nsambya HIV/AIDS clinic
tells a story of staggering need and inspirational fulfillment. The
clinic treats twelve thousand patients each year on an annual budget of about $250,000. (By contrast, almost $300,000 was spent
on my experimental transplant.) Often the money at Nsambya
doesn't stretch far enough. "We have situations where we may
run out of drugs and medical supplies," Mayanja says, sitting on
one of about thirty chairs assembled in a meeting room where
staff and patients are briefed on the second floor of the clinic.
"So, the only way out is to refer patients to private pharmacies
and drugstores. But, if a study came in that would provide medication for the study participants that would be good. So instead

of somebody getting down into their pockets to get the drugs—
or going without—then the study protocol and design would
look into that and then provide that if resources were available."[31]

The numbers, however, are only one reason why a clinical trial
would be welcome at Nsambya. It also would bring treasured resources to a place where HIV/AIDS is wreaking unimaginable
havoc, a clinic desperate for anything that can help relieve the suffering, pain, and death that touches almost every life. Mayanja, for
instance, is a trained demographer; he earned his master's degree in
demographics. His work in that field included tracking, catego-
rizing, and explicating the rates, movements, and concentrations
of HIV and AIDS in various populations throughout Uganda.
That work touched a chord because, as a child, Mayanja had been
raised by his mother's sister along with seven of her children who
became like siblings to him. Then, when he got older, Mayanja
was on hand as six of those seven each died of AIDS. "I was there
when they were sick," Mayanja recalls. "I was there when they
were being taken to hospital. I was there to give them food. I was
there to wash their clothes. So I would see exactly what went on.
One by one dying. Burying them. It taught me that the people
who are going to live, they really suffer and they need to be
helped. It's not just about numbers. It about whether they need
care, they need comfort, they need to be emotionally built up and
supported as they go through this."[32] For almost six years Mayanja
worked at the Uganda AIDS Commission, which was funded by
the World Bank. When that project ended eighteen months ago,
he was brought on at Nsambya.

Being emotionally motivated to work helping people with
HIV doesn't keep Mayanja from being cold-eyed about how
clinical trials can deliver tangible benefits to the people at his
clinic. Recently, he says, money that the clinic received to help
pay the hospital bills for critically ill HIV patients who couldn't
afford to be cared for on an in-patient basis dried up. "Now it's

either you're admitted and you will pay or we'll refer you to a nonpaying hospital with all the strings that are attached to that: the crowding, the not finding the people there, the not receiving treatment," he says with a shrug. "And that's it. Either they go without their medication or they are referred to a nonpaying hospital where they go without their medicine anyway and they go without the necessary treatment that they require."[33] If a patient was in a trial as a subject, he says, the sponsor would make sure the person was properly cared for in a hospital.

While Mayanja is open and welcoming to clinical trials participation, he is adamant that any clinical trial he would involve his patients in meet ethical standards and adhere to the tenets of good clinical practice. His boss, Martin Nsubuga, M.D., medical superintendent of Nsambya Hospital, agrees and goes Mayanja one step further. He says any trials in Uganda, and any conducted in all of Africa, should address the needs of Uganda and Africa. "If a clinical trial is going to be done right it should be designed by local scientists and Western scientists, not just Western scientists alone. It should take into account the cultural setting and the problems here."[34]

Dr. Nsubuga sees a wider potential benefit to clinical trials than just providing patients with resources and care. If Western companies or research institutions come to Uganda to conduct their trials for drugs, treatment, or devices, then it gives medical practitioners in Uganda influence over how those drugs, treatments, and medical devices are developed; it brings Uganda to the table. Dr. Nsubuga also says, however, that that doesn't give anyone license to come to Africa and conduct a clinical trial for products and treatments that Africans have no use for, such as Viagra or cholesterol-lowering medications. His position about accepting trials that address the needs of Ugandans isn't just talk or wishful thinking.

Nsambya Hospital is a Catholic-run and -supported institution.

Its full name is St. Raphael and St. Francis Hospital, Nsambya. More than two hundred thousand patients are treated per year at the hospital. The annual budget is 6 billion Ugandan shillings, or $3.75 million. "Not much by Western standards," Dr. Nsubuga says. About once a year a company or a research institution asks if they can conduct a clinical trial at the hospital. Despite the lack of money and resources that might make that yearly opportunity easy to say yes to, such inquiries are sent to an internal institutional review board, then to a second external IRB for consideration. If the trial doesn't offer help to the patients at Nsambya, chances are it's not going to get studied there. "One group was speaking to us about a vaccine for [cervical cancer] and it cost a hundred dollars each. Yes, a hundred dollars per person. That's as good as not available." Dr. Nsubuga says with a laugh. "Who can afford it? My thinking is we should factor those interests in the discussion right at the beginning. At the end it's too late. There should be some consideration for the role and involvement of Africa, which is resource poor."[35]

That said, Dr. Nsubuga and others are under no misapprehension that that's not the way clinical trials are treated at all, or even most, hospitals and clinics in Uganda. He is quick to say that ethical standards have improved and are improving, but there is a long way to go before they reach the same level as standards in place at Western medical institutions. The reason for the lag is not a lack of will on behalf of the Ugandan authorities or people and not because of ignorance about the standards. It's because of money, or the lack thereof. "When there is the promise of resources and money it becomes very difficult to think clearly," says Dr. Nsubuga, who collected consent forms from potential subjects in the microbicide trial. "This is especially true when you are running a poor institution. Sometimes the tendency is to try and cut some corners and make it easy, reduce costs and so forth. There is that tendency."[36]

Asked if doctors have to take on the role of King Solomon in balancing the needs of their patients and the lure of improving care if they help supply some willing subjects for a clinical trial, Dr. Nsubuga says flatly, "Yes."[37] In such an atmosphere the Ugandan medical establishment is wrestling with what to say to doctors who are faced with choosing to conduct a less than ethical clinical trial in order to help hundreds of sick and dying patients.

"I would say stop!" says Medi Kawuma, M.D., a British-educated professor of ophthalmology at Makerere University and the incoming chair of Uganda's Medical Research Council, which was established to oversee research into HIV and AIDS. "You shouldn't do that at all. Because we have, as you know, a protocol that should be [adhered to], especially when it's research. Especially in research when you can give a drug whose effects are not completely known, it must be very informed. It's important."[38]

Dressed in a suit with French cuffs fastened with gold cuff links, Dr. Kawuma is a formidable force in bioethics in Uganda and in all of Africa. He is the country's one and only medical bioethicist. (There is a smattering of other bioethicists in the country but only Dr. Kawuma has a medical degree.) His comparatively hard line on maintaining ethical standards comes from having witnessed a lot of questionable practices in his home country. He is a member of a committee on research and ethics at Makerere University. Each Monday postgraduate students present their dissertations on research and ethics to the committee. The section on consent, which Dr. Kawuma considers the most important part of each dissertation, is usually consigned to an appendix, and most of the time students don't present on that part because time runs out. When the committee meets to review and approve research proposals, often the members ask Dr. Kawuma for guidance on basic matters such as subject recruitment and informed consent. In one trial—testing intervention in prenatal transmission of HIV in in-

fected mothers—subjects told the research team they would be willing to take part, but only on certain conditions. One of those stipulations was that no one from the team visit them at home or at work because they didn't want their HIV status to become public knowledge. "So when these researchers see that this woman hasn't come for two consecutive visits they wait for the third time, then drive [to her home] in official vehicles that say 'HIV/AIDS research,'" Dr. Kawuma says, throwing up his hands. "No one seems to know the importance."[39]

Money, according to Dr. Kawuma, is a factor keeping Uganda from becoming the equal of Western nations in establishing and maintaining strict ethical standards in medical research. "We demand that if the United States is sponsoring research here that they should be cleared by the sponsoring country, institution, whatever," he says. "But, because of many elements the local researcher here, once they are told 'You'll be getting a thousand U.S. dollar per month,' everything else can wait. They say, 'When can we start?'"[40]

Dr. Kawuma knows that such decisions are not motivated by avarice and fulfilling personal or institutional financial need. He speaks passionately about teaching doctors and others about what is ethical and not ethical because, it seems, they just don't know the difference. "The most important thing is to educate the researchers in Uganda," he says. "They don't know what is meant by informed consent. They don't tell [subjects] they can withdraw halfway through the research. They say, 'If you tell them that then the attrition rate will be very high. We'll end up with number less than what is scientifically okay to do.' So they don't tell them they can withdraw at any time without giving reasons. They don't."[41]

This institutionalized ignorance appears to reach throughout Uganda's medical establishment. When a doctor at Nsambya Hospital is asked to make a list of clinics and research institutions in

Uganda that regularly perform clinical trials, he lists the Infectious Disease Institute (IDI) number two. Asked if he's sure about that he answers, "Oh yes. They do so many trials."[42] The IDI was founded in 2004 by a group of Ugandan and North American experts on infectious diseases and is funded significantly by Pfizer, among other groups. Asked whether clinical trials are conducted at IDI, which is part of Makerere University, Prof. David Serwadda, director of the School of Public Health at Makerere University, says that there are no clinical trials conducted there.[43] When asked why a company that doesn't sell a single drug in Uganda would help open a research institute in Uganda, Serwadda points out that Pfizer donates a lot of medication to hospitals in Uganda. He says for them it's an investment in building goodwill.[44] Pfizer, for their part, says the IDI "conducts a minimal number of clinical trials—it is primarily a health services delivery center. The institute treats patients with HIV/AIDS and other infectious diseases as well as trains medical professionals from across Africa in the latest AIDS-specific treatment and prevention options."[45] (Pfizer turned down a request to tour the IDI facilities and speak with doctors and patients at the institute.)

The atmosphere wasn't always so confused, and not every clinical trial in Uganda was as fraught with ethical danger as appears to be the case today. One of the most important discoveries in cancer treatment was made in a clinical trial conducted by Denis Parsons Burkitt, M.D., an Irish doctor on staff at the government-run Mulago Hospital, which is still the country's largest medical center. In the late 1950s Burkitt took notice of a facial tumor that occurred often on Ugandan children. The lymphoma was so severe, and at the time had few if any treatment options, that Burkitt was moved to conduct a study on the source of the tumors. He spent a minuscule grant of twenty-five British pounds on sending letters to hospitals all over Africa to figure out the distribution of the tumors. The results indicated the cause was environmental.

When he went to England to present his findings another doctor attended Burkitt's presentation almost as an afterthought. It was a happy accident because Burkitt's study helped confirm the other doctor's idea that some cancers were caused by viruses. Their collaboration led to the discovery that the cancer was caused by the Epstein-Barr virus. Another trial, in which Burkitt and colleagues covered ten thousand miles by car to further identify the boundaries of the virus, revealed that the children who contracted the tumors were set up to do so because their immune systems had been severely weakened by malaria. The clinical trials eventually led to using chemotherapy as a treatment, significantly reducing the number of child fatalities caused by the cancer.[46]

John C. Ssali, M.D., is a seventy-three-year-old surgeon, a former head of surgery at Makerere University Hospital Medical School who was also with the Medical Research Council in Uganda and is now at Kampala International Hospital. He remembers the Burkitt trials, which were finishing up in 1962 when he became a doctor. "With the success they had it encouraged people to do research here," he says. "In the 1960s and 1970s, especially, they were very active in chemotherapy research here. Looking back, there were researchers here and the research was genuine. There was genuine interest in medicine."[47]

In forty-six years as a doctor in Uganda, Dr. Ssali has witnessed firsthand how the practice of clinical trials has evolved. He has a theory about why ill Ugandans like Jackson and Annett and Charles are so easily targeted by the sponsors of unethical clinical trials: "I think we're just naive."[48] He also knows that poverty plays a role in why corners are cut in clinical trials. But it's not just the poverty of the subjects. The doctors are so badly paid that they also swell the ranks of the poor in Uganda. Although he is a committed caregiver, Dr. Ssali is not keeping office hours eight years past retirement age because of his dedication. He has not been paid his pension and so, while a lawsuit to force payment drags through the courts, he is forced to keep on working to pay his bills.

Dr. Ssali's deeper insights, however, reveal that the issues about clinical trials facing Uganda are not caused solely by some fault in the Ugandan character. The issues of ethical enforcement and doing the best for the patient, even when someone is offering a lot of money to cut corners that can jeopardize patient health, are universal to poor countries; to politically less-sophisticated countries in the third world; and to countries, like the United States, that lack government-supported medical care and base research on the demands and whims of free-market forces. "I think the time is coming for people to be inquisitive," Dr. Ssali says. "Such problems are recent. They have come with HIV infection. HIV is a new phenomenon in terms of medical history. I mean, a long time ago we had all kinds of research here and some of the topics we are discussing were not applicable then."[49]

When it comes to managing clinical trials, Uganda is facing the same challenge as almost every country in the world right now: finding a way to effectively legislate against some of the worst aspects of human nature so people can be helped and saved from disease and sickness. "There are many things which come into play," Dr. Ssali says in his slow, patient cadence. "One of them is poverty. It's greed and the poor being very vulnerable. If we recognize that it's human weakness to take advantage of the poor in this way, then we need to have laws and regulations to guard against this."[50]

He suggests a national committee on biomedical ethics in research and thinks that, given time, one will develop. "Recently," he says, "when I was on the Uganda Medical Research Council and we were traveling around the country, I would go to the medical schools and many of them were developing strong programs on ethics. I would like to hope it's going to improve."[51] On a warm, sunny afternoon in Africa Dr. Ssali would like to spend more time discussing how to improve clinical trials and ethics in Uganda, but his schedule is tight and he excuses himself to get back to work.

At Nsambya Hospital, meanwhile, Mayanja is only a few hours into his twelve-hour day at the HIV/AIDS clinic, grateful that, for now at least, he has medicine to dispense. He's aware that those drugs can run out, and he puts clinical trials on his list of possible ways to continue providing that lifesaving care.

Dr. Kawuma, at this time, is preparing to take over the MRC. He does so fully aware that battling the lure of money is a tough fight in a poor country armed only with assertions that ethical standards benefit patients when doctors can't see that direct benefit day to day. "For some the loss of one life is not much of an issue if others can continue to live and to provide better care," he says.[52] Despite that cynical assessment, he, like Dr. Ssali, sees hope. "I think we are in a formative stage. There is a lot to be done and a lot that concerns me. But, there are not many people who can see my point of view," he says looking over at Father John Mary Mooka, who is prepping for his Ph.D. dissertation on medical ethics and will come home to Uganda to practice. "I know of one man [with a medical degree] who is studying bioethics. I know there are others studying. But, to do what needs to get done, it will take time."[53] Pretty soon, Dr. Kawuma will at least be in a position to move that process forward.

Chapter 8

THE STORIES BEHIND
THE SUBJECTS

IF YOU ASK THE MILLIONS of ill people in the United States who are taking part in clinical trials why they're doing it, you'll hear many different answers, each one a personal story. Chris has hepatitis C. For thirty-seven weeks he's been taking a pill each day, part of a protocol called GI2570, half an hour before breakfast to see if it will reduce the viral load in his liver. "I don't have anything to lose," the forty-two-year-old from York County, Pennsylvania, says, "but hopefully I can gain more liver function. That's my personal goal, to see my liver heal and feel better. Trying to do something is better than doing nothing."[1]

Chris has had hepatitis C for twenty or thirty years, but it was only diagnosed four years ago and, more than likely, he contracted the incurable condition when he was nine. That was when his mother tried to kill herself and Chris found himself awash in her blood. He gets his blood drawn every six weeks, when he goes in for a scheduled checkup to track the effects of the experimental protocol. The clinical trials team also calls every three weeks between visits and gives him twenty dollars for each doctor's visit to reimburse him for his transportation costs. The side effects of the drug he's testing include flulike symptoms, aching joints, vomiting in the morning, and headaches. Neither Chris's wife nor his three children go with him on his doctor visits for the clinical trial. He trudges to his appointment, takes his medication, and adheres to the demands of the trial mostly on his own. "People have disappeared," he says about how his life has changed since his diagnosis. "People don't come around or help. People with hep C need a lot of support. It's hard."[2] To ease the isolation a little Chris, who is on disability because of his condition, is a member of an online forum where he can communicate with other people who have hepatitis C. He writes to them about his trial and his health. In addition to trying to improve his own condition, Chris also hopes taking part in the trial will help the people he meets online and those he's never met who are infected. "If none of us tried it," he says simply, "none of us would know how it would work."[3]

In a poll done for Thomson CenterWatch, a company that sells data and information about clinical trials to companies that sponsor clinical trials, the top reason people say they enroll in clinical trials is to find "better medical treatment" (although whether that means for themselves or others is not made clear). The second most often given reason is to help advance medical research.[4] Mike falls into that category.

Mike is a forty-year-old artist living in New York City. When he's not busy meeting with clients to work out the details of their photography and illustration projects, Mike is at the NYU/Bellevue Hospital Center testing an experimental vaccine for HIV. After an initially intense round of screenings, Mike, who is not HIV positive, received monthly injections of a modified adenovirus, which is similar to a virus that causes the common cold but is masked to appear as HIV in England's body to see how the potential vaccine reacts. After three months Mike was put on a schedule that brought him to the hospital, at First Avenue and Twenty-seventh Street, once every six months, where he is tracked as part of the study. He will continue to make the trip twice a year until 2011.

"If I could be one of five or ten thousand people who can

help millions of people, that would be great," Mike says. "I tell everybody about it, to raise awareness. Plus, yes, it's part pride. I'll do what I can to help, I'm proud of that."[5] Mike says that no one should get busy starting a campaign to make him Saint Mike because—and this does not diminish his altruism—at the beginning of the trial his motives were not utterly selfless.

"My ex-lover, who was HIV-positive, and I went into the trial together," Mike says, "and the upshot was we were able to have sex the way we wanted. The assurances we received in our testing from the trial let us have a better relationship."[6]

Mike's enrollment in the trial has opened his eyes to a little-appreciated phenomenon taking place in the gay community regarding HIV and AIDS and, in turn, has stirred his desire to be active in HIV/AIDS prevention. He says he's noticed that people in the United States are not as careful as they once were in their sexual practices. "There's a vigilance fatigue at this point," Mike says about why he is so vocal about his participation in the trial. "Young people think it's an old person's disease. That's simply not true."

Mike's father, who is an administrator at a homeless shelter in Miami, is impressed that his son is enrolled in the trial and is trying to help others. When Mike told his doctor about the trial he was curious and asked a lot of questions. Other people are impressed when Mike tells them what he's doing. Then there are people who lecture him about the danger of testing an experimental drug; they insist, Mike says, that all clinical trials are bad and that he's putting himself at great risk. "Sure, it could be dangerous," says Mike. "But I can't see why I wouldn't do this. I'll do whatever I can."[7]

Some people say polls that try and explain why subjects choose to enroll in clinical trials are not reliable. When given a choice people will tend to provide the more flattering answer than the more self-serving answer to just about any question. The reason most people enroll is to get what they perceive as better medical care than they can get through standard treatment. "I think people are out there looking for a treatment that gives them some greater chance of symptom relief or cure depending on what their condition is," Dr. Paul Appelbaum says about why people enroll in trials. "They've come to see clinical trials as a way of achieving that."[8]

Dr. Ezekiel Emanuel interacts with thousands of clinical trials subjects yearly at the NIH's Dana Farber Institute, a hospital dedicated to conducting only clinical trials. He finds that many subjects are motivated to enroll for a single reason. "If I'm sick my focus of interest narrows considerably . . . Once you are sick you have one goal: to get better."[9] But, he says, that's not the end of the story. In clinical trials, helping others is closely connected with helping oneself. "Many people enroll for different reasons. Chief among them is to get some benefit. Another is to express your altruism. Most people want to get a benefit, yes, but, in cancer trials, the number two reason overwhelmingly given for enrolling in trials is that people want to benefit other people down the road."[10]

Sandra Burks is intimately familiar with why people enroll in clinical trials. An attractive, enthusiastic, hardworking, and experienced registered nurse, Burks is associate director of the Surgical Therapeutic Advancement Center at the University of Virginia Health System. She runs a research office offering cardiac patients clinical trials options after surgery. She is overseeing twenty clinical trials right now. Burks also has been a patient coordinator in clinical trials for almost twenty years. She even took part in a clinical trial studying how to cure the common cold when she was an undergraduate at the University of Virginia. They put her and other students in a hotel over spring break, exposed them to cold viruses then took notes on what happened to each student.

Her job as a patient coordinator means that she deals with the nitty-gritty logistics of supporting subjects in clinical trials. She will answer their phone calls and their questions, assist in physical exams, get prescriptions filled, deal with insurance companies, act as a go-between for doctors and subjects, and take care of all the little and large issues that need to be attended to on behalf of subjects. "I tell new coordinators that a large part of their job is minutiae," she says. "We love to be problem solvers. We get an issue for a patient or a group of patients and we figure out, 'How do we solve for this?'"[11]

While the job is not glamorous, it is rewarding. "The best part of my job is seeing the end of the data, when we can answer a question," Burks says. "It's really cool when it turns out the way we wanted it to. It's good to be connected to patients over a long period of time and then to see those results that can help them."[12]

Conflicts have to be negotiated before the rewards can be reaped. "Sometimes people sign up for a trial for, say, a new device," Burks says. "They want the newest device, but it's a randomized trial and sometimes they don't get the new and improved device. I try to explain that to them beforehand. Sometimes they really understand, sometimes they still think they'll get the device."[13]

She describes therapeutic misconception as a widespread issue and a cause for concern in her field. She acts as a nurse and patient advocate and can only make sure that each subject is well informed about what it means to be a subject. The way each subject thinks about the trial, whether as treatment or research, is really up to each subject. "I have a lot of respect for the fact that each trial is not designed primarily to help people," Burks says. "That's a sacred trust, to inform patients about the difference between research and treatment. But I'm hoping it will help them. You can't take that hope away from people."[14]

Burks isn't talking about hope only in reference to subjects seeking treatment for themselves through a trial. People will volunteer for a trial because their condition is genetic and they don't want their children to suffer. Some volunteer because a relative has the condition being studied and they want to help.

Still, some subjects come in with great expectations, and if the trial proves more challenging or uncomfortable than they thought it might, they drop out. The term for it is "loss to follow up." Burks respects a subject's choice to drop out. Even though gathering data and research is the goal of every clinical trial, the safety and comfort of subjects is not forgotten. It is her job, and the job of other patient coordinators, to make sure information can be derived from subjects while at the same time they are kept informed and safe. "In health care people are a lot more informed than they once were," Burks says. "Patients are having a lot more opportunity to participate in clinical trials. They should be taken care of after they make that decision."[15]

Sister Mary Andrew Matesich was president of Ohio Dominican College (now University) for more than two decades, a dedicated scientist with an M.S. and a Ph.D. in chemistry, and a subject in four clinical trials investigating treatments and cures for breast cancer. Her journey as a subject captivated the interest and admiration of thousands of people and was the focus of media coverage throughout the country, most notably in a front-page story in the *New York Times* and a profile by Betty Rollin on PBS.[16]

"I am a scientist myself," said Sister Mary Andrew. "The scientist in me was interested [in clinical trials]. As a sister, a member of a religious order, someone in a service capacity my whole life, I want to continue to be of service to others. I wouldn't be alive today if other women hadn't been in clinical trials."[17]

Sister Mary Andrew looked at clinical trials as a way to achieve a legacy that would transcend her pain and sickness. "As long as I can be helpful with trials, I'll do it," she said at a time when her cancer continued to spread. "I'm not really looking for a cure. I'm going to die of this disease, I know. It's a way of having that death be more meaningful."[18]

While media reports focused heavily on her devotion to helping others by enrolling in trials, that wasn't the only reason Matesich was so willing a participant. A devout woman of God, Sister Mary Andrew was utterly truthful in explaining her motivations. She said it felt good to wage a fight, to take action, against the disease ravaging her body. She also said it gave her hope, and she believed, despite the very long odds, she stood a chance for recovery because she was trying everything possible. "You have to realize that the chances of something spectacular happening are very slim," she said, "but not impossible."[19] Sister Mary Andrew died peacefully on June 15, 2005,[20] having done all she could to transform her suffering into something good for herself as well as, most notably, for others.

Once a subject enrolls in a clinical trial their number one concern is personal convenience rather than the level of care, the safety, or the risk associated with whatever drug or treatment they are receiving.[21] Specifically, 54 percent of subjects surveyed said they wanted to make sure their appointments could be scheduled so they weren't too inconvenienced; 46 percent were worried about risk, and the same percentage of subjects said they were most worried about the side effects of what they were testing. Crunching the numbers even further, 31 percent of subjects interviewed were concerned that the investigative site for the trial be accessible by public transportation and just more than 20 percent wanted to make sure their office visits were kept to the lowest number possible.[22]

One doctor said that based on his experience, he was highly doubtful about whether subjects, as polls showed, were more interested in advancing science than they were in their own treatment. He said, for instance, that often subjects are so focused only on their own care that it is common for them to lose interest and stop showing up for scheduled appointments or tests without notifying anyone on the research team.[23] However, he is quick to add, there certainly are brave and dedicated subjects enrolled in many trials.[24]

Lori Ratliff is a nurse who has been a patient coordinator involved in clinical trials for more than a decade at UVA. Through her job the fifty-year-old from Ivy, Virginia, has worked intimately with subjects in clinical trials. For everything from recruiting and answering questions to helping manage prescriptions and finances and more, Ratliff was the person subjects called for help in negotiating the demands of a trial. But in June 2004 Ratliff found out exactly what a subject goes through in a clinical trial when, as part of one, she became the first person in the state of Virginia to receive an islet cell transplant to cure diabetes. (She received the transplant and was the first subject in the UVA trial in which I subsequently enrolled.) Her unique, dual perspective as simultaneous subject and researcher makes it easy to understand why when Ratliff talks about the unsuccessful transplant she received, she says, "Oh, it was worth it. It was a disappointment to me, but I think it helped UVA evolve into a much stronger place for trials."[25]

Ratliff says as a patient coordinator she becomes "enmeshed in people's lives. You become their social worker, their primary care person, everything. You have to be this person's support system."[26] Manning those front lines of research, Ratliff knows firsthand that the lines between treatment and study in a clinical trial are "very fuzzy."[27] When she agreed to be the first person on board as a subject in UVA's islet cell transplant program Ratliff honestly didn't do it so she could get better treatment for her condition. "I had no expectation it might work," says Ratliff, who has lived with type 1 diabetes for thirty-two years and suffered from life-threatening hypoglycemic unawareness before the transplant. "It was such a foreign concept to me to not have diabetes. I never considered that I might not have it. When it became an opportunity right here there was no question I would do it because it was such a great opportunity for UVA."[28]

Eleven days after seven hundred thousand cadaver islet cells were infused into Ratliff's liver, UVA announced that the state's first islet cell transplant procedure was a success.[29] Ratliff was taking half the amount of insulin that she had been before the transplant, and there was hope she might one day be insulin independent. However, just two months later in a development that Ratliff says "came out of left field and surprised everyone," she developed antibodies that started attacking and killing the new islet cells.[30]

"The immune system is a complicated thing," Ratliff says. "Before the transplant my tests for antibodies were in the acceptable range, and they thought I wouldn't produce cells that would harm the islets. But, after the transplant it turned out there were obscure antibodies that were a result of my having been pregnant years before."[31] Ratliff was given the choice of dropping out of the clinical trial as a subject. If she did it would mean that she could stop the punishing regime of immunosuppressant medication. She chose to stay on the drugs and endure the side effects until the research team could figure out exactly what went wrong with her transplant.

Six months later, when a lot of information had been collected from her, Ratliff chose to go off the antirejection drugs and drop out of the trial. "For me personally," she says, "the most amazing thing was when I was three months into the study and taking the immunosuppressants. It was very difficult. The side effects were very hard to tolerate. I was relieved when I came to the decision to stop. It wouldn't have helped the trial to stay enrolled and that was important."[32]

After stopping the immunosupression, another unexpected thing happened. Although not "cured," or insulin independent, Ratliff was still benefiting from the transplant. She was taking less insulin than before the transplant and she no longer had severe hypoglycemic unawareness. "It's been a huge gain for me," Ratliff says, "and for UVA. Although it was a disappointment that we didn't get the expected outcome, we learned something. And that's what this is all about."[33]

Quite a lot of attention is rightly paid to the rights of subjects in clinical trials. In international agreements such as the Helsinki Declaration and the Nuremberg Code there are specific protections for subjects. The rights are so widely understood and accepted they are even spelled out by companies when they try and recruit subjects. Subjects must be fully informed of the risks of the trial and give fully informed consent to enroll. They can stop participating in any trial at any time for any reason. They can say "no" at any specific time to any research procedure being done to them.[34] What, though, are the responsibilities of subjects enrolled in trials? Do they have an obligation to be as informed as possible about their particular trial and about trials in general?

"An obligation? No," says Dr. Emanuel. "They only have an obligation to protect their own self-interest."[35]

Others are not so sure about the scope of subject responsibilities as Dr. Emanuel. Some bioethicists say that as a social compact every generation owes it to future generations to become subjects in clinical trials and develop lifesaving treatments and drugs. One prominent bioethicist, Arthur Caplan, gets a little more specific in arguing that all people who receive care at a research or teaching hospital incur an obligation to be subjects in clinical trials because they are benefiting from the care they receive at a research institution. Going to a teaching hospital, where doctors are frequently accompanied by medical students, residents, and others when they perform exams, is already a de facto agreement to be a research subject, Caplan argues. He stops short of saying everyone who gets care at a teaching hospital must enroll in a clinical trial. It is, in his view, a theoretical argument about an existing social obligation and not a manifesto for people who received care at research hospitals.[36] It's also a view not held by a majority of bioethicists or doctors. Most come down in the middle between a subject's obligation being nonexistent and being mandatory.

CSL Behring, a biotherapies company that produces blood-related products, is up front and clear about what responsibilities subjects in their clinical trials bear. During the informed consent process the company insists that before the start of the trial subjects become well informed about the study, the team conducting the study, even the facility where the study will be taking place. They ask that subjects understand what will be expected of them and commit to fulfilling those expectations. They urge subjects to write down concerns and ask as many questions as possible about anything they might not understand. Once the study is under way CSL Behring says that subjects should tell any other doctors they see that they're enrolled in the study, should inform the trials team about any side effects they may be experiencing as a result of the study, and should inform the study team if they are hospitalized or need emergency medical assistance for any reason while enrolled in the study.[37]

There is no specific data on whether the majority of subjects follow such advice. There is one study that sheds a little light on how seriously subjects take clinical trials in general, and it doesn't speak well for the awareness and acumen of those who sign up for experimental treatments.

In a study to find out what subjects enrolled in clinical trials for cancer treatments thought about conflicts of interest, such as researchers or hospitals paid by the same sponsors of clinical trials being conducted by the hospital or researcher, 90 percent say they're not worried about it. In almost every conceivable additional scenario presenting a financial conflict of interest between drug companies and researchers the majority of cancer sufferers were not bothered by the conflict: 77 percent of patients said they still would have enrolled in the trial if their cancer treatment center owned stock in the company sponsoring the trial; 81 percent thought it was ethical for researchers to be paid speaking fees by the sponsors of the clinical trials they were working on; 70 percent would have enrolled even if they knew beforehand that the researchers conducting the trial owned stock in the company sponsoring the trial.[38] Fewer than half the subjects wanted to be told about what kind of oversight was in place for conflict of interest issues or wanted disclosure of any financial ties between researchers and the companies sponsoring trials.[39]

And the questions were not about some theoretical possibility. They were about a real and growing problem in clinical trials research that compromises subject care. Researchers getting money from a company and doing a clinical trial for that company are less likely to act in the best interests of the subjects than they are to act in the best financial interests of the company and themselves. It isn't as if such things rarely happen. "A survey of hospital review boards that act as watchdogs for experiments on patients shows that one in three members take money from companies that make drugs and medical devices that come under study," the *New England Journal of Medicine* reports. "What's more, many of those with conflicts [of interest] rarely or never disclose their financial ties, researchers found."[40]

Why didn't the subjects care about something that potentially affects their care directly? It's not that they were poor or ignorant. The people surveyed were, for the most part, educated, financially stable, and white.[41] They were also more concerned with getting the best care possible—which they thought was available only through clinical trials—than they were with side issues such as conflicts of interest. Most subjects were focused primarily on curing the cancer they suffered from and thought collaboration between researchers and drug companies made a medical breakthrough more and not less likely. Finally, the study hinted that subjects who are seriously sick, such as people suffering from cancer, care a lot more about getting better than they do about who might be getting rich trying to come up with a cure for cancer.[42]

Out of a deep financial need fifty-year-old Gail Ogden, of Westmoreland, Kansas, has been caught in the bind between what clinical trials subjects owe to science and what science owes to subjects. When Ogden was diagnosed with hepatitis C she discovered she couldn't afford the cost of drug treatment even after her insurance paid for part of it. Suffering from liver damage and very sick, Ogden listened to her doctor's advice and volunteered as a subject at the University of Nebraska in a forty-eight-week-long clinical trial. The trial was testing a hepatitis C treatment, called Rebetron, against treatment with two drugs, ribavirin and interferon, to see which lowered the liver's viral load more effectively. The trial was sponsored by Schering-Plough, a drug company.[43]

Ogden was accepted into the trial and was assigned to take Rebetron. The drug has some serious side effects, such as tiredness, fever, and depression so severe that some people who take it seriously contemplate suicide. She intended to stay in the trial until she knew whether or not the drug was working and lowering the viral load in her liver. If it wasn't working then she planned to drop out. She didn't get the chance to make that decision.[44]

Almost two months into the study, with the side effects so intense that she had to leave her job on disability, Ogden asked the trial's sponsor for the information on her viral load. The company said no. They told her they were withholding the information about how well the drug was or was not working until the trial ended. They chose to do so specifically to keep people from dropping out of the study. "I had no idea the extent these people would go to get their drugs to the market," Ogden was quoted as saying. "It's absolutely disgusting, the corporate greed in America."[45]

A spokesperson for Schering-Plough, Robert Consalvo, says the step was taken not to pad corporate profits but because keeping the information from subjects would help retain subjects and that would contribute to making sure the trial was successful. Also, he says, patients are not trained or expert enough to decide on their own to drop out of a clinical trial based on medical test results. While those arguments are compelling, Consalvo really hit the nail on the head by saying that being a subject in a clinical trial is not the same as being a patient treated in a doctor's office. He also adds that perhaps sponsors of clinical trials need to do a better job of making subjects aware of that difference.[46]

"Sick people can't think of themselves as research subjects," says Dr. George Annas, the specialist in health and law at the Boston University School of Public Health. "They don't want to feel like they're being used as guinea pigs. They want to feel like patients. But they're not. They're guinea pigs."[47]

Despite her outrage over being treated like a "lab rat," Ogden is sticking with the study. As she says, "It's the only chance I have.[48]

It's not only sick people reaching out for any cure or chance at hope by enrolling in a clinical trial. That intense desire for results no matter the risk can spread to people close to whomever is sick, especially if it's a child. Dave and Lynn Frohnmayer, of Eugene, Oregon, started an entrepreneurial fund to try and develop new treatments for a rare disease that was threatening to take the life of their twelve-year-old daughter, Amy. The inherited disease, called Fanconi anemia, is a rare condition that destroys the bone marrow cells that produce red blood cells and is the result of a faulty gene. For the Frohnmayers, the disease had already taken the lives of two daughters, Katie at age twelve and Kirsten at age twenty-four. When Amy was diagnosed the Frohnmayers decided they would do whatever they could to find a cure. The problem was, scientists were barely able to decipher the cause of Fanconi anemia much less find the cure.[49]

Dave Frohnmayer, who is president of the University of Oregon, started the Fanconi Anemia Research Fund, Inc., when he realized the dearth of information that existed about the disease. Raising $6 million, the fund at first focused on experimental gene therapy to attack the condition.[50] The idea was to explore introducing a functional gene into the system of a Fanconi anemia subject to replace the faulty gene that was causing the anemia. "I have no doubt that gene therapy will be one of the major advances of early twenty-first-century medicine because so many disorders can be attacked by this method," Frohnmayer says. "This will be . . . a tidal wave within the next ten to twenty years."[51]

The Frohnmayers also established summer camps for children with Fanconi anemia, interested researchers in investigating the disease and dispensed funding, put together a scientific review board, and in 1988 held a conference with eighteen scientists and a few patients.[52]

All the money and the test-tube research led to initial limited testing in a clinical trial. Lynn Mendenhall, who at forty-five was the oldest person to be living with the condition in the United States, underwent experimental gene therapy as the first step on the path to curing Amy's anemia as well as her own. "If I were in her shoes," said Mendenhall, who was suffering from cancer as a result of Fanconi anemia and who was close to Amy and her family, "I would be scared to death . . . I think about her a lot. I want this gene therapy thing to work so bad because I don't want her to go through this."[53]

Mendenhall lived for five months after receiving the experimental gene therapy, and died from cancer. The gene therapy had no impact on her condition and did not contribute to her death.[54] The fund continues its work, and one of its top priorities is to further clinical research to cure the three hundred or so people who have Fanconi anemia in the United States.[55] The odds are stacked against being able to launch full-scale clinical trials specifically for Fanconi anemia patients because so few people suffer from the disease. Instead, results from trials for other conditions can be extrapolated and applied to solving the complicated riddles of the disease. The fund, however, is helping support clinical trials that have significantly improved the rate of successful bone marrow transplants to extend the lives of people with Fanconi anemia, says Mary Ellen Eiler, the executive director of the fund. "That means now patients are living longer than they were previously, some into their twenties."[56] One of those is Amy Frohnmayer, who is currently enrolled at Stanford University.[57]

Joe Giffels talks to hundreds of people on a regular basis about clinical trials. He talks to subjects, patients thinking about becoming subjects, and just regular people curious about clinical research. He blogs about clinical trials on WebMD, giving advice and information about trials and covering everything from Graves' disease and migraine studies to how FDA regulations protect subject rights. It's something he is uniquely qualified to do as assistant vice president of academic affairs and director of research integrity at the University of Maryland, Baltimore, with degrees in chemistry and biology, and a former administrator for an institutional review board. Despite his forum, Giffels says most people don't know much about clinical trials.

"Trying to write or inform people about clinical trials is very difficult, I find," Giffels says. "Most mainstream media are not that interested in the topic. Big pharmaceutical companies are not at all interested in giving candid answers about research. And I'm amazed, with the millions of people in trials, that the federal government hasn't set up a specific set of rules just for clinical trials so people are better informed."[58]

Part of the problem with reaching people en masse with information about trials might be because they are, in Giffel's words, "a very diverse group who are all motivated by so many different things like money, treatment, helping others. Overall though, I'd say most people enroll because they're going along on this wave. A doctor will recommend a trial to a patient during treatment and they'll get caught up in it and think of the possibilities and they'll want to do it."[59]

As far as whether most subjects are primarily motivated to seek treatment for themselves or to help others, Giffels comes down squarely in the middle. "I think the majority of people want to contribute something, but they also want to be cured at the same time," he says.[60]

Giffels has written movingly in his blog about subjects who have died in clinical trials. He informed people about a unique legal case where it turned out the blood, tissue samples, and other materials a subject provides researchers in a clinical trial were found to be the legal property of the researchers and not the subject. He wrote clearly about pending FDA regulations for clinical trials and urged readers to provide any comments they had to lawmakers before the regulations were enacted.

On his message board Giffels gets many questions such as those asked by family members of subjects about side effects from a drug trial, by subjects about dropping out of a trial if they want to, or wondering if they can't sleep because of the medication they're taking for a trial they're enrolled in. But he overwhelmingly has to answer a single question: "99.9 percent of the time I am asked 'Where can I sign up for a clinical trial?' "[61]

While Giffels thinks most people consider clinical trials a treatment option and not some researcher's idea of what might possibly work, he also thinks people are able to access more tools than ever before to be in charge of their own care in a trial. "The downside," he says, "is that people have to do a lot of Web surfing and research on their own to find information. That's why I always tell them to speak up when they are with the researcher in the trial. Ask questions. Ask about new data on risks and side effects. People are medically savvy, I think, but that doesn't matter if they don't ask questions."[62]

In contrast to the history, horror, and headaches of some clinical trials, most run uneventfully and produce positive benefits for the subjects enrolled and for people in general. Wendell Steele, a sixty-six-year-old native of Harrisonburg, Virginia, knows first-hand what it feels like when everything in a clinical trial goes according to plan.

Before he had surgery to remove a cancerous tumor from the top lobe of his right lung, he was asked to participate in a clinical trial. "I did some checking and spoke to the people at the hospital, the people involved with the trial, and my own doctor and said yes," Steele says.[63]

The National Institutes of Health was sponsoring the trial to develop a way of cutting down on the recurrence of cancer in subjects after surgery. Half the subjects would receive postsurgical chemotherapy while the other half would not receive chemo. Steele says he had no idea which group he would be in when he signed up. He agreed to do it because his sister Elaine had died of cancer and another sister, Janet, was battling ovarian cancer, and he wanted to contribute and help others. It turned out Steele was in the group receiving postsurgical chemotherapy.

The sponsor of the trial, however, was not going to be paying for the chemotherapy. That was left to the trials' subjects. "My insurance covered the treatments," Steele says. "If they hadn't I wouldn't have done it. I wouldn't have been able to."[64] With that squared away, all Steele had to negotiate were the intense side effects of three sessions of chemo, which in some people, such as his sister Janet, includes diminished appetite, nausea, and hair loss.

After successful surgery, Steele drove the two hundred or so round-trip miles to Charlottesville once a week for three sessions of chemotherapy spread out over a month. Luckily, the chemo never made him nauseous or took away his appetite for his daily snack of cheese and crackers, although his hair did thin out a little. He agreed to go back for checkups to track his progress once every six months.

"Apparently it helped," Steele says in his soft southern accent about the results of the trial. "All my checkups were clear. I feel it definitely helped me."[65] And Steele's participation definitely helped others.

Two years into the trial they stopped recruiting new subjects. The trial was declared an early success and shortly afterward, short rounds of postsurgical chemotherapy became standard treatment for lung cancer patients. Several years later Steele still makes the trip to Charlottesville once every six months for follow-up checkups. He is still enrolled in the clinical trial, and he is still cancer free.

As mentioned previously, Jesse Gelsinger wasn't so fortunate. His father, Paul, a Tucson resident, says Jesse was the kind of kid you wanted to strangle one minute and hug the next. "He could crack you up and make you mad at the same time," Gelsinger says. "Jesse was a pistol growing up. He was more than a handful. Of the six children, Jesse was definitely more work than all the rest combined."[66]

Besides his boisterous personality, what also made Jesse a handful was ornithine transcarbamylase (OTC) deficiency syndrome, the condition he suffered from as a young child. By the time Jesse was eighteen years old he was taking a relatively new medication that reduced his OTC to a mild form of the disease. To return the favor of benefiting from such an effective medication, and because he was told he could help children suffering from OTC, Jesse volunteered for a clinical trial at the University of Pennsylvania to try and develop a cure through gene therapy. "He wanted to give back and he wanted to help," Paul Gelsinger says. "I mean, it was about helping babies. He could potentially be helping himself someday by advancing the technology. But there wasn't going to be any direct benefit to him, and he understood that and I understood that."[67]

Jesse checked into the hospital for several days of extensive screening and tests before undergoing a surgical procedure as part of the trial to cure OTC. The surgery involved placing one catheter into his hepatic artery, at the inlet to his liver, and another at the organ's outlet to monitor the blood as it flowed from the liver. An experimental viral vector that was designed to increase the efficiency of enzymes that metabolized protein was infused into Jesse's liver. It was hoped that the vector would boost Jesse's efficiency from a paltry 6 percent. To determine the results of the procedure, researchers would do a liver biopsy one week after the infusion.

Immediately following the procedure Paul Gelsinger received a call from the trial's principal investigator who said Jesse was fine, that he was recuperating, and that he'd only have some flu-like symptom for a few days. That came as a relief to Gelsinger, considering the rigorous surgical procedure Jesse had gone through. Gelsinger was proud of his son for weighing the risks and rewards of the trial and deciding to take part. He had been alongside his son every step of the way helping him examine the risks. In fact, when the principal investigator first called Jesse to say he had been accepted into the trial, Jesse asked the investigator to call back to talk to his father about it also. The investigator called back and talked to Paul Gelsinger about early results of the trial from other subjects. He thought they sounded extremely promising. Even though he was working as a licensed handyman, Gelsinger has considerable expertise and experience in science and chemistry from his days spent as an engineer and technician for Dupont and Mobil. He had become very well versed on OTC in order to care for his son when he was a young child.

When the investigator reeled off technical information that included percentages of response to the vector in mice, monkeys, and other human subjects, Gelsinger grasped the importance right away. "He brought up that the most recent patient had showed a 50 percent increase in her ability to excrete ammonia after the treatment," Gelsinger says recalling the conversation. "I said, 'Wow!' Literally, I said 'Wow!' I said with Jesse's ability at only 6 percent then you might be able to show exactly how well this works. And he said yes and said it would be for the benefit of these kids. With that kind of information, how do you not help?"[68]

Both Jesse and Paul Gelsinger were also told on the phone and in the consent form that there were risks. Jesse could contract hepatitis from a liver infusion. His chance of death was put at one in ten thousand. The Gelsingers were told, however, that the greatest risk would come from the liver biopsy one week after the surgery to measure the results. After carefully weighing the pros and cons and going so far as to seek out the opinion of an independent OTC expert at the University of Arizona, Paul Gelsinger had backed his son's decision to become a subject in a clinical trial.

On Tuesday, one day after Jesse's surgery and after being told his son was fine, Gelsinger began receiving more calls from the hospital and in each call the news about his son grew worse. On Tuesday evening Gelsinger was on a plane from Tucson to Philadelphia and arrived Wednesday morning. By the time he walked into the hospital to see his son, Jesse's condition had deteriorated to the point where he was in a coma and on a ventilator. Jesse rallied then worsened. Thursday morning doctors told Gelsinger that his son's organs were shutting down one by one, that he had suffered irreversible brain damage, and that they wanted to disconnect him from life support. Numb and in shock, Gelsinger nonetheless started making calls and gathering family members. Soon Jesse's room was crowded with aunts, uncles, cousins, and ten people from the hospital staff, along with the principal investigator for the clinical trial. A chaplain delivered a final prayer and while family and friends stood with their heads bowed, Paul Gelsinger looked up and signaled it was time to stop the ventilator and the other machinery keeping his son alive. The principal investigator of the clinical trial then placed his stethoscope on Jesse's chest before saying, "Good-bye, Jesse. We'll figure this out."[69]

Gelsinger was told his son's death was a tragic, horrible, unforeseeable accident, the result of the price one pays for pushing the boundaries of science. In the months after his son's death, as controversy and blame for the tragedy swirled, Gelsinger publicly and privately supported the investigators on the clinical trials team. Six weeks after Jesse's death one of the principal investigators in the trial was even present when Gelsinger scattered his son's ashes on a mountain in Tucson.

Around the same time the OTC expert from the University of Arizona told Gelsinger something he hadn't been told by doctors and researchers before the trial: Monkeys had died testing the same vector used on Jesse, albeit in lower doses. The expert urged Gelsinger to start looking into how well the FDA was overseeing the trial. Gelsinger discovered notes from a meeting in 1995 when the FDA and the NIH, apparently reacting to pressure from "industry," pulled the plug on a project to establish a database for sharing information among researchers about adverse reactions in gene therapy clinical trials.[70] Gelsinger still withheld any judgment, but he was getting suspicious because things didn't seem right with the trial.

In December 1999 Gelsinger met for the first time with James Wilson, M.D., the head researcher on the trial, to review the results of Jesse's autopsy. While sitting together on Gelsinger's back porch in Tucson, Gelsinger asked Wilson if he had any financial interest in the outcome of the clinical trial. Gelsinger later alleged that Wilson said he was an uncompensated consultant for the biotech company, Genovo, which was developing the gene therapy treatment tested in the trial.[71]

Later in December Gelsinger agreed to go to Bethesda, Maryland, for a conference of medical experts reviewing the facts surrounding his son's death. A day before the conference he was also scheduled to visit Dr. Wilson at the University of Pennsylvania and talk to members of the clinical trials staff. On that trip, while awaiting a connecting flight, he spoke on the phone with an executive at the FDA. He told the executive that at the conference, which would have media present, Gelsinger intended to be vocal about the FDA's oversight lapses in his son's trial. The next day the FDA put out a news release placing the fault for Jesse's death squarely on Dr. Wilson's research team. "It seemed I had really touched a nerve in those guys," Gelsinger says.[72] He became more concerned with the kinds of information coming out about his son's death but still supported the doctors on the research team.

The next day, at the conference in Bethesda, Gelsinger was told that the efficacy of the treatment tested in Jesse's trial had never been proved before his son took part. Contrary to what Jesse and Paul Gelsinger had been told, there was never any indication that the treatment Jesse was testing worked. "I was just so upset," Gelsinger says. "I was devastated. I had trusted these men. I already had the information that these guys had violated the protocol, that monkeys had died, and that they treated Jesse when his ammonia was too high. They had admitted to me his ammonia was too high. But that last piece of information was the straw that totally broke my back as far as being able to support these guys. And I couldn't support them anymore." Gelsinger got a lawyer. Shortly afterward more disturbing revelations came out:

- The lead researcher at the University of Pennsylvania involved with the trial, Dr. Wilson, had a direct financial interest in the success of the trial.
- A nurse who was the informed consent witness when Gelsinger signed the consent form resigned from the trial ten days before Jesse died over concerns about the trial, including that her questions about side effects were not being answered. She never informed anyone about her worries at the time.
- Less than 10 percent of adverse events in all gene therapy clinical trials using viral vectors similar to the one Jesse received had been reported to federal authorities, contrary to regulations.[73]

One year and one day after his son died, Gelsinger filed a lawsuit against the three principal investigators, the University of Pennsylvania, and the institutional review boards responsible for monitoring the clinical trial. (He also wanted to take the FDA and other government agencies to court. "The FDA had the [adverse event] information and didn't disseminate it," Gelsinger says.[74] Federal agencies, however, have immunity from such lawsuits.[75]) The lawsuit he was able to bring was settled for an undisclosed amount in just six weeks. The settlement didn't heal all the wounds, though.

"We never got any justice out of this," Gelsinger says. "I mean, we got financial compensation in the form of a lawsuit. The Department of Justice did an investigation and ended up essentially giving these guys a slap on the wrist. After a three-year probationary period, they let them go back to work. They were not fined personally. Their institutions were fined. So these guys basically got told you did wrong but we're going to retrain you and you get to go back to work."[76]

Gelsinger was dissatisfied with the deal as it was struck. "You know what we wanted? We wanted the documents related to what happened. We wanted the findings that they uncovered. We wanted those released to the public so the media could have access to it. And we wanted a public apology from the principal parties in this for their actions. We wanted a public acknowledgment of wrongdoing and we wanted an apology." Asked if he got either, Gelsinger says, "No. I told the Department of Justice that for those reasons, I could not support their settlement. I wasn't asking for jail time, I wasn't asking for money. I was just looking for nothing more than what we should have gotten. We didn't get those things."[77]

After the Justice Department's investigation, and after Gelsinger testified before a congressional committee examining his son's case, he started speaking at medical conferences several times a year. "Jesse's story needed to be told. The general population probably has very little awareness or understanding of what my son did," Gelsinger says. "But the research community knows who Jesse Gelsinger is and they see him as a benchmark in the ethical development of clinical research. His case is a signpost. It's a place people can go to, and stop, and see where an awareness change happened."[78]

He bears no personal animosity toward the investigators involved in his son's death. "I . . . don't think they're bad men. I've never felt like they were bad men. They were just men who got lost. They became blind and they got lost in their own ambition. And my kid died as a result of that, as a result of a system that failed to keep that ambition in check."[79] Neither is he unilaterally against clinical trials. "I'm not opposed to clinical research," he says. "I never have been. I'm opposed to unethical clinical research. Big difference."[80]

But in recent years Gelsinger stopped going to conferences and speaking about Jesse. While he thinks there is a heightened awareness of issues in the medical community, he says those changes haven't been translated into significant ethical reforms; he believes what happened to his son can happen again.

In 2007 Gelsinger stopped giving presentations because it became too painful. "Because of the way he died, you can imagine the impact that had on me," he says. "He was doing exactly what I tried to teach him his entire life, which was the proper way to be. And here he demonstrated that for me and died doing it. That's a tough thing to carry, and he left it for me to carry. He was a hero for volunteering, for putting himself out there for other people. Isn't that what a hero is?"

While the legacy his son left for researchers and subjects involved in clinical trials is still being decided, the positive impact, as a person, that Jesse had on his father resonates loud and clear. "If [Jesse's] looking down he would probably say, 'Get past it. This is something bad that happened, move past it.' I'm trying to move past it."[81]

Chapter 9

TRANSPLANTED

WHILE I WAS on the waiting list to receive pancreatic islet cells that would be implanted into my liver as part of a clinical trial to cure type 1 diabetes, I had to see an endocrinologist on a regular basis, have a tissue typing blood test repeated, and visit a pulmonologist at the University of Virginia. A nodule had been discovered in one of my lungs during a chest x-ray that was part of the screening process to see if I would be a candidate for the clinical trial. I was hoping the pulmonologist at UVA would say the lump in my lung was a simple benign growth and clear me to continue as a subject in the trial. The first time I went to see him he reviewed the tests that had already been done on my lung, performed some more tests, and notched up the suspense by telling me he'd let me know. A few weeks went by before I got a call to come in and see him. I sat in the doctor's office quietly and expectantly on the paper-covered exam table, waiting while he was looking at the test results and murmuring. Finally he said he agreed with my pulmonologist that the nodule wasn't cancer. But, he said, it could be benign or it could be fungal or bacterial. He couldn't recommend that I remain a subject in the clinical trial. I was done.

He was making his recommendation because he wasn't sure what the nodule was. MRIs and CT scans could only show what the nodule looked like, the shape and texture, not what it was made out of.

What about a biopsy? I asked. He told me that would mean taking a needle, jamming it into my chest through my lung into the nodule, taking out a piece, and looking at it under a microscope. Okay, I said. The pulmonologist said no to that kind of test because needle biopsies are not 100 percent reliable and the trial required absolute certainty about my health.

The UVA pulmonologist wasn't out to deny me a chance to cure my diabetes. He was only looking out for me. If I had the transplant and it turned out the nodule was bacterial or fungal, once they put me on antirejection drugs to suppress my immune system, the bacteria would be free to run rampant throughout my body. He was doing the best thing for me, really. Before leaving I asked if I had *any* options at all. He said offhandedly that I could always have surgery to have the lump removed. If they did that they would not only know what it was, it would be gone.

I asked him to tell me more. The surgery would mean collapsing my right lung. Once the lung was collapsed the lump would show itself, like a foot sticking up under a bed sheet. They would perform laparoscopic surgery to remove the nodule along with part of my lung. Once they removed the nodule, they would culture it in a lab to determine for sure whether it was fungal, bacterial, or inert. The surgery would require three days in the hospital and a two-week recovery at home.

The surgery was routine but still risky because, after all, it was a lung. A few days later I told Winsor, the patient coordinator for the clinical trial, that I was considering having the surgery. She made it clear to me that neither she nor anyone on the clinical trials team was advocating that I have the surgery. It was completely my call.

Two powerful forces made up my mind to do it. The first was

money. I got a new job and my old, affordable, comprehensive, wonderful health insurance was set to expire at the end of April. If I waited until then to have the surgery, under my new insurance, I would have to pay thousands of dollars out of pocket.

My other motivator grew out of how for years I had successfully waged a daily battle with diabetes; but no matter how hard I fought and kept fighting, I knew I would never win. The best I could hope for was to keep playing defense against a condition that would eventually kill me. Now I had a chance to go on offense. Even if it didn't work, I knew I would regret it forever if I didn't at least try.

I checked into St. Mary's Hospital in Richmond for the surgery in mid-April, almost thirteen months after I first heard about the clinical trial. Afterward my doctor described the surgery as "uneventful." I told him that for me, it was a pretty big event.

For two days in the hospital I had a chest tube draining fluid from my lung. Once they removed the tube and ran tests, I was discharged. I went home for two weeks of recovery, which meant going stir crazy and listening to Traci tell me not to do too much. A week later I saw my pulmonologist for my follow-up visit. He was thrilled with his work and with how great I was doing. He said he used ninety-eight titanium staples to put my lung back together. I saw the little rivets on my x-ray. They were looking great, the surgeon said. And no, he told me, the staples wouldn't set off metal detectors at airports. After that visit, it was another waiting game for a definitive answer to what the nodule was.

Three weeks later I found out it was fungal. That meant the surgery was, in the end, a good idea. If I had gone on immunsuppressants with the nodule in my lung, it could have caused major complications.

Like Hercules seeking penance through his twelve labors I had vanquished yet another restriction. A few weeks after the surgery I felt fully recovered. In no time I was back running five miles a day. I was fit, rested, and ready for my transplant, ready to get the clinical trial going and get those islet cells producing insulin in my liver.

Then, just like when limited grant funding threatened to make the trial too expensive for me, everything again came to a screeching halt. The protocol for the study had to be updated because of changes in requirements dictated by the FDA. Winsor reassured me that when the clinical trial started up again, I would be the first person in line to receive a transplant. There was, however, no estimate on how long the trial might be idle. It could be a few months, even longer, she said. Hercules never had to deal with the FDA.

I continued with my job and when I finished the New York City Marathon in November, I tried to ignore how much better I might have done if I hadn't been hit with hypoglycemia a few times during the race. If the transplant comes through, I thought, that will not be a problem in my next marathon. That's when something occurred to me. I had run five marathons as a diabetic. What if the transplant worked and I didn't have diabetes? What were the possibilities? That's when I started making plans to run a fifty-mile race after the transplant.

It wasn't until another year after my lung surgery, the following March, that Winsor called me to say the new protocol for the trial had been revised and approved. I asked her if that meant we were back on, if the clock was ticking for me to have the transplant. She said not quite. I needed to have a few tests run again because it had been so long since they conducted the evaluation. Then another problem came up. The endocrinologist caring for me at UVA was questioning whether I was suffering from hypoglycemic unawareness sufficiently enough to justify the risk of receiving the transplant.

This new obstacle caught me completely off guard. My previous medical records showed that I had spent a fair amount of time having seizures, passing out, and going into multiple comas from hypoglycemic unawareness. However, in the three years that I had been using the insulin pump, I had only been taken to the hospital in an ambulance twice and paramedics were only called to my house once. That, apparently, did not qualify as severe hypoglycemic unawareness to the endocrinologist. The pump, she said, seemed to have solved the problem.

On top of that, the endocrinologist had concerns about whether I fully appreciated the risks of participating in a clinical trial that, like all clinical trials, might not provide me with any benefit at all—in fact, it might harm me. She thought I was a little too eager to get the transplant. She interpreted my eagerness as an indication of a defect in my comprehension of the risks posed by the clinical trial and of the strenuous regime of continuing care and maintenance that would be required of me after the actual transplant.

I volunteered to write a letter to a review panel explaining why I thought I should be in the clinical trial. The doctors on the clinical trial team thought that was a good idea. They also said I would have to undergo a complete neurological/psychological evaluation by UVA psychologists to determine whether I was cognizant enough to understand that the trial would demand a lot from me; that it had substantial, long-term risks; that it might not be successful; and that it might harm me.

I shared my outrage over the situation with a friend of mine. He told me he could see their point. Having a chunk of my lung removed to stay in the study, he said, seemed a little "extreme." That made me think carefully and objectively about whether I was on too much of a crusade with the trial. I decided I wasn't being unreasonable. I was just a subject enrolled in a clinical trial, which is a bit like the medical version of extreme sports. My clinical trial, more than most other trials, was by its very nature, risky and dangerous. But making progress in the fight against diabetes required going to extremes. Later I said to my friend, "Extreme? If someone told me I had to light my hair on fire every day to cure diabetes, I would do it."

I wasn't that blunt when I met with the psychologists for my neuro/psych exam. We spoke about the generalities of the trial and what I thought about the risks. Then I took a bunch of standardized tests where for forty-five minutes I associated words and compared apples to more apples in diagrams. Two weeks later, the panel reviewing my participation in the trial had a meeting. They discussed my tests, my letter, and my psychological profile. Then they cleared me to continue in the trial. My name was put on the organ donor list with no restrictions. Now I just waited for the call that a really generous person with a big pancreas and my tissue type had died.

People ask me whether I think about the islet cell donors. They ask if I want to meet their families so I can thank them for how much their loved ones did for me. I answer that I don't. I feel that act of contributing something so precious, of being so generous at the time of a loved one's death, is an act I can only repay by making the most of the gift they gave. The only other thank you I can contribute is to encourage everyone to do what I have done: Sign up to donate your organs so others can live better, longer lives.

The call came on a Saturday afternoon. They'd found a matching donor and were prepping the islet cells for transplantation at the University of Pennsylvania before they were shipped to UVA. They would perform the transplant the next day or perhaps Monday, if everything went according to plan. It was May 13, three days after my forty-first birthday. Traci and I packed a bag and hit the road to Charlottesville.

The General Clinical Research Center where I had had my overnight evaluation was closed for admittance on Saturday so I was put in what I called the hospital's "general population." That night and into Sunday, Traci and I were lucky to have a nurse who looked the other way and let us snuggle together in bed. Throughout the next two days the anesthesiologist, an endocrinology intern who was assisting, and several other doctors came by to talk to me, explain procedures, and run tests. All of these serious-minded medical professionals who usually behaved in a calm, officious manner with their patients were as enthusiastic as children about the procedure. They smiled at me and talked about how amazing this was, how I was on the cutting edge of medicine, and how they hoped they would get a chance to see the procedure performed. In short, they were stoked. I finally appreciated why I had been treated like a medical celebrity when I had showed up for my evaluation eighteen months earlier.

Monday was the day of the transplant. That morning they wheeled me to the GCRC wing. They hooked me up to an IV of immuosuppressants called thymoglobulin, which is derived, believe it or not, from rabbits and commonly used to suppress the immune system before transplants. I had woken up Monday with a splitting headache and feeling sick to my stomach because my blood sugar had gone down to 49 the previous night, so it wasn't a great day to start with. Then things got worse.

I had a severe reaction to the thymoglobulin. I developed a slight fever that eventually shot up to 104.7 degrees. By the middle of Monday afternoon and into the early evening I thought I was dying—not that I felt like I was dying or wanted to die, but that I was actually dying. I had to stay on the immunosuppressants in order for my body to accept the islet cells. Dr. Brayman gave me steroids and switched me to a different IV immunosupressant called Zenapax, which they hoped would be gentler on my system.

Everyone waited to see how well I tolerated the new immunosuppressant. Doctors, ready to go and dressed in surgical gowns, came in, checked on me, and stood around. I tried to will my fever down. I couldn't accept that after all it had taken to get to this point we would be stopped. It was like some cruel joke.

Traci asked Winsor and Michael Hanshew, who would be replacing Winsor when she moved on to a new job she'd gotten, about my reaction to the thymoglobulin. They said it happened sometimes, but what was going on with me looked particularly severe. At seven thirty that night Dr. Brayman came in and took my temperature. It was down around 100. I was wiped out but glad to hear some good news. It was time to decide whether to go ahead or wait for another time and another donor. He asked me if I wanted to try for it.

I believe I said, "Hell yes!" He said there was some cause for concern, but he felt it was safe to do the transplant, even with the slight fever. Traci didn't look completely convinced. Dr. Brayman put his hand on my shoulder and told us both that when he counseled patients on decisions such as this one, he tried to think about what he would do if he were the patient. "I also think," he said, "about what I would do if the patient were my brother, or my wife. I think it's safe." We decided to go ahead with the transplant.

A team of nurses and technicians came in and spent twenty minutes wiring me up with tubes and electrodes for the surgery. By the time they were finished I looked like a cheap stereo. Before the operation one surgeon said I had nothing to worry about, that he had done an infusion before. Before the procedure Dr. Brayman showed Traci and me a translucent plastic pouch containing yellow sludge. I held the bag of islet cells in my hand then posed for a photo with Dr. Brayman, Traci, and the insulin-producing cells that would go into my liver.

The actual transplant took less than an hour. They ran a tube into my portal vein through a small incision, poured the cells in, and put a plug in to seal the incision. By midnight I was back in my room watching David Letterman with my wife.

The next morning and afternoon I lay in bed disconnected

from my insulin pump waiting to see what would happen. Dr. Brayman came in and checked on me. I had little red spots all over my feet that freaked out Traci and me. Dr. Brayman seemed puzzled and intrigued by them. He wasn't sure what they were but said not to worry, they might simply be a side effect of the medication I was taking. He and the team would keep their eyes on them. More important, to me, was that my blood sugars were running high. I asked Dr. Brayman if this was bad news. Did it mean the islet cells aren't working? On the contrary, Dr. Brayman said it was good news. The cells were alive. If they had been rejected they would have died, dumped their insulin, and sent my sugar low. Now it was just a waiting game. The cells would take their time setting up in my liver and when they were ready, would start producing insulin. Or not. In the meantime, I would go back on my insulin pump, try not to tire the cells out, and see what happened. There was no strict game plan for adjusting my insulin doses if the cells came online. I would have to play it by ear.

The red spots cleared up in a few days, but I still left the hospital as a walking, talking science experiment. Like every other subject in a clinical trial, what would happen next was anybody's guess.

To give the cells a rest I couldn't run for the next two weeks. Instead, I spent several hours twice a week before work for the next month driving to LabCorp to have my blood drawn, and driving back and forth to Charlottesville four times in the next two months for hour-long doses of IV immunosuppressants. I began taking heavy doses of Rapamune and Prograf, oral antirejection drugs that were among the twelve pills I took every day. When I wasn't busy with that, I was keeping detailed daily logs of my medications, my food, my exercise, and my overall health. It was like having a second job. Traci created a binder and designed special forms to keep track of all the notes and paperwork. We put my bottles of medications in a plastic grocery bag and hung it

from a doorknob in the kitchen. Because I was on more pills than Elvis, I found it necessary to assemble my doses into plastic daily organizers each Sunday night for the week ahead rather than pick through all the bottles in the bag every day.

At the same time we were busy with this in Richmond, the clinical trial team in Charlottesville would keep very close tabs on how I was doing and decide whether I would need another transplant. They would keep me on the transplant registry and might give me another infusion if cells became available and they thought I needed them.

The antirejection drugs made me tired and gave me so many canker sores in my mouth—at one time more than a dozen—that for a while I couldn't eat because of the pain. When my tongue also swelled up significantly the drugs were cut back for a few days.

A month after the transplant, on my own I decided to not give myself the usual dose of insulin before lunch that kept my sugar from going high. I wanted to see what might happen. Like many diabetics I routinely adjusted my insulin doses to accommodate fluctuations in day-to-day activities and diet that impact blood sugar levels. After lunch my blood sugar spiked to 287 but over the next few hours it came down on its own, with no insulin. It dropped about 100 points in two hours. The transplant was working.

Then, in June, I felt like I might be catching a cold. With my compromised immune system I worried that the sniffles could progress into some sort of raging infection that would destroy the islet cells. Traci and I weren't sure what to do. Should I not leave the house? Should I dose up on vitamin C? Do I increase or decrease my meds and, if so, which ones and by how much? Before doing any of those things, Traci suggested I call Michael Hanshew and tell him what was going on. He said Dr. Brayman would be interested in hearing about this. I called Dr. Brayman's office and spoke to a nurse about what was happening. I expected her to take the message, speak to Dr. Brayman, and call me back with specific instructions if there were any. Instead the nurse put me through to Dr. Brayman while he was in the middle of surgery! I felt silly interrupting him while he was transplanting someone's kidney to tell him I thought I might have a cold. On the phone he dismissed my worries and said to keep my meds where they were and to go immediately to an emergency room if I developed a fever. Otherwise, there was nothing to worry about.

The next day I woke up coughing, vomiting, and dizzy. I didn't have a fever but it was time to make a visit to the emergency room at Retreat Hospital, an institution that had been built during the Civil War. They popped a saline IV into my arm and let it drip for a few hours, checking on me from time to time. They seemed to be out of their depth. After a few hours they called Dr. Brayman, who instructed them to have me transported sixty miles by ambulance to UVA Medical Center. I watched out the back window of the ambulance as Traci trailed behind us in her pickup truck for the hour-long drive to Charlottesville. After two days in the hospital my condition stabilized, I got over whatever bug I had caught, and I went home

Aside from that bit of drama, things settled down. Two months after the transplant my insulin requirements leveled out at forty units a day, which was half of what I was taking before the transplant. I was still on my insulin pump and we kept a bag packed in case I got a call that there was another donor. Traci and I almost grabbed that bag twice when it looked like a pancreas had become available to provide more islets for a second transplant. Each time, though, it was a false alarm. I worked closely with Michael Hanshew, and my antirejection drugs were closely monitored and adjusted. I got a prescription for a lidocaine mouthwash to numb my mouth and relieve some of the pain from the sores caused by Rapamune, one of my immunosuppressants, but they couldn't prescribe anything to give back the energy the medication sapped from me.

I was looking forward to the three-month, post-transplant mark in August when my meds would be cut back significantly and I would require fewer blood tests and trips to Charlottesville for checkups and IVs. I hoped I would begin to feel like myself a bit more. It had been a tough experience. It wasn't only the side effects of the drugs but also the constant monitoring, record keeping, and wondering and worrying about every minuscule little symptom.

In late July Michael asked if I would speak with a potential participant in the clinical trial and tell him about my experience. He said I should be completely truthful when Marcus called me and to simply answer any questions he had. I was happy to do it. The success of the trial would depend on recruiting more participants, and I knew it was difficult to find qualified candidates who were also willing to endure the arduous nature of the trial. I also thought it was important that whoever did become involved in the trial knew exactly what they were getting into.

Over the phone with Marcus I shared how good it felt to be able to fight back, finally, against diabetes. I told him the staff members on the clinical trials team were responsive, competent, caring people. Marcus had a lot of logistical questions about the time commitment, how much the medications cost if they weren't covered by insurance, how often I had my blood drawn, and other practical considerations.

I told him one thing that made the trial manageable on a day-to-day basis was that my wife, Traci, and I were involved in every aspect of the trial together. She went with me to every doctor's appointment so we could talk about it afterward, share notes, and get a better perspective on what happened. She would research things I would have never thought to consider, then ask Dr. Brayman or Michael about them when we went to appointments. Her involvement, however, only went so far and she could only offer so much help. I knew that was difficult for her. There were times I felt tired and annoyed from all the medication or from having to wake up at five A.M. to drive to UVA or LabCorp before work for a fasting blood draw or an IV or a checkup every few weeks. Sometimes I got short-tempered and frustrated from the record keeping and the sheer volume of work that went into continuing in the trial. Traci could only sit there as I screamed at traffic while driving, angry not because someone didn't use their turn signal but because the day-in and day-out slog and grind of the trial took a toll that went beyond pills and blood sugar fluctuations. I told Marcus that despite my misplaced tantrums, I was glad to be in the trial. I said there was no way I could be in the trial without my wife by my side.

Marcus said he had loving, strong-willed family who would help him the same way Traci was helping me. He thanked me for my time and for answering all his questions. He said he had a decision to make. I wished him luck. He eventually decided not to enroll.

Just when the three-month post-transplant window was about to close, when I could start training for the New York City Marathon in November, and when the intense regime of medications, blood draws, and clinic visits would be eased back, they found another donor. On August 1, Traci and I spent our second wedding anniversary in the hospital prepping for another transplant, which I received the next day.

The second time around was much smoother and easier; the miraculous had become routine. Every member of the transplant team performed flawlessly without even much comment; they transplanted 850,000 more islet cells into my liver, then sent me home in two days. For the next three months I was on the same

punishing schedule of care I had just completed. I worked with
my endocrinologist to adjust my insulin as my need for it kept going down. I was disconnected from my insulin pump in September. I was taking a single injection of ten units of insulin a day. I
kept sticking my fingers and testing my blood sugar up to six times
a day. I kept expecting my blood sugar to soar but it didn't.

I couldn't ever remember not taking insulin, not worrying
about my blood sugar rising or falling. I couldn't recall not having a juice box in my glove compartment or LifeSavers (I se-
lected them for the name) in my pocket in case my blood sugar
went low. Now, when I was tired or ate too much or felt light-
headed from standing up too fast, I paused and thought with absolute awe, "This is what regular people feel like." If I had a
presentation to deliver at work and was nervous about it beforehand, I thought, this is only what it feels like to be nervous and
shaky, not hypoglycemic and shaky. Throughout my entire life if
I felt light-headed, I tested my blood sugar. If I felt sluggish and
tired, my first thought was that my blood sugar must be high.
Every physical sensation I had was put in the context of diabetes.
Now for the first time I knew what everyone else felt like. It was
all new and amazing and miraculous.

I even made a small bit of history in September when I became the first, and to the knowledge of my doctors, the only person in the world to have received an islet cell transplant from a
donor with a blood type different from mine. My second donor
had type A blood; I have O positive. The discrepancy was not
caught when the cells were processed in Philadelphia then sent to
UVA and infused into me. It wasn't that drastic because while
organs must match by blood type, bone marrow and other cellu-
lar transplants are not blood typed. Until my case, it was part of
the protocol of the study to match the cells by blood type. I was
assured that the problem wouldn't have any medical effect on my
transplant. I was told that it might even change the protocol so

that subjects and donors did not have to be matched by blood type. Like most medical discoveries, it was an accident that might prove beneficial.

Some less trivial news hit that same month when the *New England Journal of Medicine* published the results of a study showing that islet cell transplantation might not live up to the promise of being an applicable cure for diabetes. Out of thirty-six subjects who were studied, 86 percent of them were back on insulin two years after their transplants. That meant that only five subjects were still off insulin. The odds, it appeared, were stacked against me. But so far I was on a roll. I was sure I would be in the 14 percent who would make the transplant work. No study was going to dampen my belief in a bright future.

By October I was taking only four units of insulin per day. That small dose acted as an immuno-buffer to keep the islet cells from being too stressed. Four units was nothing, really. A nondiabetic person could take four units of long-acting insulin a day and it wouldn't do anything to them. As far as Dr. Brayman and I and the team were concerned, I was insulin independent, or as good as cured.

That fall Traci and I were invited to a football game at UVA with Paul Manning, the man who funded a large part of the study with his own money. We sat in a skybox and met his two incredible children, who were in college, and his wife. It was gratifying for us to show Manning where his investment went. I also met with other potential financial donors who might give to the transplant program at UVA to try to persuade them that they should contribute generously to expanding the Pancreas Islet Cell Transplant study at the hospital. I testified before a state legislative committee in support of having Virginia fund stem cell research programs to further, and eventually perfect, the kind of research started with me. I was interviewed by a television news reporter about the success of the Pancreas Islet Cell Transplant trial at UVA. I was happy to help spread the word.

In November, with the second three-month cycle of clinical visits completed and the medication and doctor visits finally cut back to a manageable schedule, I got back to serious running with the idea of completing a fifty-mile race in a year. That January I started a four-month training program to complete an April marathon as a training run.

Throughout the early winter I noticed that I felt hungover and battered from the previous six months. Now that the most intense treatments were in the past it was like I was suffering from post-traumatic stress. I chalked it up to just that—stress brought on by going through a very tough medical adventure. Traci was in grad school working hard for her degree in occupational therapy. I was running and writing and working and, while things were not difficult, I was flat out tired from the efforts of the previous year. Traci suggested I see a counselor to help manage my moods, and I said that I would get over it. I said I was simply adjusting to things having been difficult. It was natural . . . it would pass. I expected my old, enthusiastic self to return with the spring and looked forward to running a marathon without having to lug around my insulin pump.

In early March, just to see if I could do it, for one week I completely went off insulin. The first day I ate a ham sandwich and my sugar didn't go up. It worked. I was walking a tightrope without a net and I wasn't falling. I sent an e-mail to Michael and Dr. Brayman confessing my accomplishment. Dr. Brayman congratulated me and told to get back on four units of insulin a day to safeguard the long-range health of the cells.

One Saturday in March, almost three years after I first heard about the clinical trial, I ran twenty miles with no blood sugar problems at all. It was on that day that I felt like I was finally seeing the payoff for all the work, as though I were emerging at long last from a tunnel and into the light. I was face-to-face with a future that looked more promising than it ever had before. I had gone through a struggle, persevered, and emerged better for it.

The next day after breakfast Traci told me that for many months it had hurt her to see me in so much pain from my medical problems, that she didn't believe those problems would ever be resolved, and that she didn't want to be married to me anymore. She moved out that day and just like that, our marriage was over.

I told Dr. Brayman a few days later what had happened. He said he had seen marriages end before when a chronically sick person became well. He said he was initially shocked but not totally surprised. I, on the other hand, would remain stunned over my wife's sudden departure from my life for countless months.

To lift my spirits a bit, Dr. Brayman invited me to a fundraiser dinner for the Juvenile Diabetes Research Foundation. He introduced me around the room, and then had me stand up before the entire ballroom full of people as an example of what research can accomplish. While we were waiting for the dinner part of the evening we both met a man who had received an islet cell transplant five years earlier and was still off insulin. I thought to myself that whatever the *New England Journal of Medicine* said, that would be me in five years and beyond. The clinical trial had cost me a lot, more than I ever bargained for, but there was still a lot to gain, there was still history to be made. For the first time since Traci walked out I felt a little better about the future.

Then a few weeks after my marriage suddenly failed, the islet cells in my liver ever so subtly began to fail. That was when I learned what it really meant to be a subject in a clinical trial.

My insulin doses crept up slowly. In May 2007, on the one-year anniversary of my first transplant, I was taking ten units of insulin a day. Five months later, in October, I was taking twenty-five units of insulin a day. The increase, I was told, could be attributed to stress in the months following the breakup of my marriage and from making plans to move back to Arizona. Tests showed that I was still producing insulin and the islet cells appeared to be healthy. I was told it was a wait and see game. There was no reason to panic. When the stress eased, once my divorce was final and I was back home and settled into a new life in Arizona, the cells could return to their previous level of effectiveness. I packed a U-Haul trailer and drove across the country to Arizona in November with plans to fly back to Virginia for a scheduled checkup in February.

By January 2008 I had split my insulin dose and was taking fifteen units in the morning and another fifteen in the evening. It wasn't much more insulin than I had been taking months earlier and things appeared to be holding, or at least not getting worse. Then over ten days in late January and early February, the roof completely fell in. My blood sugars started going very high after I ate anything. Normal blood sugar is between 85 and 120. One day I ate a bagel and it was like I ate a chocolate Easter bunny. My blood sugar spiked to 345. I took fast-acting insulin to knock the high sugar down. Nothing happened. I took more. Still nothing. After a third dose, it backed down to 230. Clearly something was wrong.

Over the next nine days the same thing happened again and again and again. I kept notching my insulin up, both fast-acting when I ate and long-acting in the morning and at night. Lying in bed each evening I imagined I could feel the islet cells dying. In the morning and throughout each day I would shoot more and more insulin into myself like I was pouring sand into burlap bags to hold back a flood. I had to keep the stress off the remaining islet cells. I had to get my blood sugar under control. I had to get through this. By February 3 my blood sugars stopped rising—I was taking a morning and an evening dose of long-acting insulin every day, plus I was injecting fast-acting insulin four or five times a day, usually before eating anything. On February 4 I dug through some boxes and found my old insulin pump. I put it in my desk drawer and started preparing myself to begin wearing it. Once again, I was an insulin-dependent diabetic.

Before flying to see Dr. Brayman at UVA I sent him a detailed report on how my insulin needs had increased. He wrote an e-mail back saying, "Yikes!" and promised a slew of tests would be run to find out what exactly was happening with me.

On Friday, February 8, I sat in an examination room at UVA with Dr. Brayman and Courtney Garbee, the new patient coordinator on the study. I was told one option that might help me was to reduce my immunosuppression dose. That might actually lower my blood sugar because one effect of the medication was that it raised blood sugar. Dr. Brayman also said they would look at taking me completely off immunosuppression. That would mean I would be out of the clinical trial. Without thinking I said, "If it's going to help you to keep me on immunosuppression, then keep me on it. If you can get information from me for the study, even if I have diabetes, then I want you to keep getting information from me." I have no idea why I said that. It wasn't my intention. It wasn't part of any plan. But those were my sincere wishes. At that moment, I realized that the clinical trial was more important than just what I could get out of it. The study was important. If not for me, then for someone else. Dr. Brayman said they would look at the test results before making a decision but they would do what was best for me.

A few weeks later my immunosuppression doses were reduced. My insulin requirements remained the same. My status had changed: I was now an insulin-dependent diabetic enrolled as a subject in a clinical trial to cure diabetes that, at least for a little while, had been successful. Later that month I was driving to the supermarket with my cousin Daniel. I was feeling sorry for myself.

I was complaining about having to take all these drugs, plus insulin, and how I felt like I got screwed. I did a few minutes of "Why me?" while Daniel listened. When I finally stopped he looked at me, shook his head, and said, "Dude, look at what you did. Look who you may have helped. Look at what you contributed. That's worth something."

Of course, he's right. It took years of effort, the loss of my marriage, and the end of my "cure" for me to fully come to terms with the fact that when you are a subject in a clinical trial you're rolling the dice. You hope you'll win but, even if you don't, you hope someone else will gain something from your participation. I am hoping that in the other areas of my life I can be as genuinely giving and generous as the people who donated their cells to me. I am hoping I can live a life that rises above mere self-interest.

One day in April 2008 I forgot to take my morning dose of long-acting insulin. Throughout the day my blood sugar didn't go inordinately high. I took my evening dose as usual. The next day, I started my own little clinical trial by skipping my morning dose of insulin. Again, my blood sugar was stable throughout the day. I stopped my morning dose permanently, effectively cutting my insulin dose by half. Just like that. My doctors were happy for me but couldn't explain why this was happening. I didn't count on the trend returning to where it had once been when I was insulin free. If that happens that would be great. If it doesn't happen, that's great too. Either way, I'm still in the fight. I'm still able to say, "At least I tried."

Afterword

VOLUNTEERING FOR
A CLINICAL TRIAL

IF YOU'RE THINKING of volunteering for a clinical trial there is some information you should keep in mind.

BEFORE YOU DECIDE TO ENROLL

1. Volunteering for a clinical trial is a legitimate option you might wish to consider if you're seeking a new way to address a medical condition you have. However, clinical trials are not medical treatment. You might benefit from a trial, but that is not the reason the trial is being done. The trial is being conducted to gather data—period, end of story. Never forget this, it will help you manage your expectations. Be honest with yourself about the possibility that you might not benefit from the trial and that you might even be harmed. Make a list of pros and cons about your decision and talk it over with those close to you to see if it's the right decision for you. Also, research all possible treatment options for your condition before opting for a trial. Ask your doctor, get a second opinion, and scour the Web and resources at the library for information from reliable sources about possible treatment options you might not be aware of.

2. Volunteering for a trial to help others and advance medical science is honorable. Many people feel compelled to "give back" or

to sign up for a trial exploring new treatments and drugs for a condition a family member or loved one suffers from. If such an option feels like something you want to do, then by all means consider it. Before diving in, however, conduct thorough research at the library or over the Internet to learn as much as possible about the area of medicine the trial you're considering is addressing. Talk to your doctor and people close to you about the pros and cons of your decision. Never sign up for a trial on a whim and without first doing proper research. If your gut tells you to volunteer, wait a few days or longer and see if, after proper consideration, you're still as passionate as you were when the idea first occurred to you.

3. Finding a clinical trial is not difficult. There is a very comprehensive listing of more than fifty thousand open trials prepared and maintained by the National Institutes of Health at www.clinicaltrials.gov. The listing isn't sponsored by a company or group with a self-serving interest to recruit subjects, so it's a trustworthy resource. You can search trials by condition, drug intervention, location, and sponsor. Another good listing site is www.centerwatch.com, a for-profit information services company that serves the clinical trials industry. These, and other sites, are completely free. There is never a legitimate reason to give any personal information or pay a fee to any listing service. (The same holds true for the actual trial. No legitimate trial will ever charge you to take part. Some might incur financial commitments for medications, tests, etc., and those must be revealed before you consent to take part.) Also ask your doctor if any trials in your area of interest are being conducted near where you live or by someone he or she recommends.

CONSENT AND QUESTIONS

1. When you first visit the sponsor of the trial, find out the full name of the person with whom you are speaking. Ask them to describe to you their role in the trial. They could be a nurse who has very little information about the trial; or they could be the patient coordinator, with whom you will work closely during the course of the trial; they might even be the principal investigator, who is in charge of the trial. If the person doesn't seem to know a lot about the trial, which may happen in your first meeting, ask for the name of someone who has more specific information so questions you have can be addressed.

2. For your first visit (and for subsequent visits) take someone with you. This is helpful because you are going to be receiving a lot of information and it's often difficult to process it all on your own without having someone to review it with you. Ask the researchers if the person with you can accompany you through all aspects of your visit, including an exam. This is helpful because you might only be hearing "cure" or "treatment" while the person with you is hearing "side effects" and "risk." If the person can't be with you at all stages, that's fine, they'll be immediately on hand following your visit so you can discuss what happened while it's fresh in your mind. You might also bring a pad and take notes, or even a tape recorder, to capture what was said for you to review later on.

3. Informed consent is crucial to the clinical trials process. It is a federal regulation that you give informed consent before the trial. **If you are not offered informed consent along with an informed consent form to review and sign before you take part in the trial, do not take part in the trial.** Before signing the informed consent form you will be told in person and in writing the risks and benefits of the trial, what you will be

expected to do, what the trial is for, and many other specific aspects of the study. According to the Office for Human Subject Protection at the University of Rochester Medical Center, here is what you should be told:

- That the trial involves research
- The purpose of the research
- How long the trial is expected to take
- What will go on in the study and which parts are experimental
- Possible risks or discomforts
- Possible benefits
- Alternatives to the research treatment that are available
- That the FDA and others may inspect the study records, but the records will be kept in a confidential manner
- Whether medical treatments may be available if you have side effects, what the treatments are, where you can get them, and who will pay for them
- Who you can contact with questions about the trial, your rights as a research subject, and injuries related to the research
- That being in the trial is voluntary and that you can quit at any time without otherwise affecting your treatment or the services you receive.[1]

During this time you can ask questions. Don't be bashful. Ask about anything you are the slightest bit unsure of or unclear about. Questions you should ask include:

- What exactly is going to happen to me during the study?
- What are the side effects?
- Will the study provide free treatment for any side effects or ill effects of the trial?

- Will I benefit personally from the research?
- Can I leave the study at any time?
- What options other than taking part in the study do I have?
- Will taking part in the study cost me anything?[2]

Ask for the opportunity to take the consent form home to study and discuss it with others. If it's not possible to take it home, it's a good idea to have someone with you at the visit to help review the form before you decide to consent or not.

Take the advice of Paul Gelsinger and ask a member of the research team to give you any adverse events information from the trial or from other locations where the same trial is being conducted. Also, ask for the name of an expert in the same field being studied who is not involved in the trial so you can contact that expert and ask his or her opinion.[3] You can also find an expert on your own who is doing research in the field of the trial. Before I consented to my trial I called an endocrinologist who used to treat me and who was a diabetes expert I trusted and asked him about islet cell transplantation, about the university that was conducting the study, and his opinion about the procedure. It was extremely helpful in making my decision to pursue the trial.

DURING THE CLINICAL TRIAL

1. At any point during the trial you can drop out. This is a guaranteed federal and international right. While not necessary, it is good etiquette to let the research team know that you are dropping out and, if you feel comfortable sharing the information, the reason you are not continuing.

2. Be sincere about your involvement. Keep a diary if it's required. Go to all appointments you agreed to go to. Take all the

tests you agreed to take. Adhere to the guidelines you agreed to when you signed up. This is important to ensure accurate data from the trial. More important, if you have an adverse reaction and you did exactly what you were asked to do each step of the way, you and the research team can be more assured of its origin and pinpoint whether it's a result of the trial.

3. Continue to ask questions. You should ask and expect answers to questions about the clinical trial overall, about your test results, about results thus far from the trial, about side effects, about what to expect in the next step or steps in the trial, and about anything else that you are not clear about or that you are merely curious about as you proceed through the trial.

4. Ask the research team to copy your primary care physician on all your test results. Let your primary care physician know you are asking this and to expect these test results. This provides an independent review of your results and will inform your own doctor of any drug interactions or other effects from the trial that may impact your overall health care.

5. Take an active role in the study. You are a partner in the research and as such you should continue to research the area the trial is studying and the progress of the trial and related studies. You should keep a diary (even if it's just occasional, it's better than nothing) of what is happening to you during the trial, missed medication doses, or anything and everything you think might be relevant to the research team or just as notes to yourself to keep track of what's going on. Make a binder or book to keep records, test results, the consent form, contact names and numbers, and other information for easy access. This is also useful to share with other doctors you see for care during and after the trial.

6. Ask the sponsor or the patient coordinator for the results of the trial as it progresses and when it's concluded. Knowing exactly what's happening and what happened is important for your own peace of mind. It's also valuable to be able to share the information with doctors you might someday see because the trial may impact your health in the future and should be taken into consideration when you receive care.

ACKNOWLEDGMENTS

Thank you to the following people for helping me research and write this book:

Dr. Kenneth Brayman
Richard Byrd
Elizabeth Caspar
Kendall Davis
Ed Dumas
Jennifer Edwards
Jeremy Fischer
Paul Gelsinger
Al and Jo Hart
Jeff Kellogg
Kathy Mayle
Father John Mary Mooka
Lisa Marie Morrison
Stephanie Nolen
Traci Steele

Jackie Johnson, my kind and patient editor at Walker & Company

and Joy Tutela, my talented and thoroughgoing agent at the David Black Agency

NOTES

INTRODUCTION

1. Adil M. Shamoo, "Death by Research," *Webdiary*, 2006, http://webdiary.com.au/cms/?q=node/1501, accessed July 14, 2008.
2. Ibid.
3. Robert Fee, "The Cost of Clinical Trials," *Drug Discovery & Development*, March 01, 2007, http://www.dddmag.com/the-cost-of-clinical-trials.aspx, accessed July 14, 2008.
4. Author interview with Paul Gelsinger, February 14, 2008.
5. Alan Fischer, "Tucson's a Hot Spot for Clinical Trial Drugs; Experts: Ethnic Diversity Here a Big Plus," http://www.tucsoncitizen.com/ss/frontpage/54121.php, June 6, 2007, accessed July 14, 2008.
6. N. R. Kleinfeld, "Diabetes and Its Awful Toll Emerge as a Crisis," *New York Times,* January 9, 2006.
7. Ibid.
8. Ibid.
9. Becton, Dickson and Company, "Blood Sugar Diary," BD Getting Started™, 3.

Chapter 2: THE RIGHT AND WRONG OF CLINICAL TRIALS

1. Author interview with Dr. Paul Appelbaum, March 13, 2007.
2. Shirley Telles, R. Nagarathna, and H. R. Nagendra, "Breathing Through a Particular Nostril Can Alter Metabolism and Autonomic Activities," *Indian Journal of Physiological Pharmacology*, 38, no. 2 (1994): 133.

3. Donald G. McNeil Jr., "Vaccine to End Cervical Cancer Conquers Myths—and a Virus," *New York Times/International Herald Tribune*, September 12, 2006, http://www.iht.com/articles/2006/08/30/healthscience/snvaccine.php, accessed July 14, 2008.

4. Richard Twyman, "A Brief History of Clinical Trials," The Human Genome (a Web site sponsored by the Wellcome Trust, a British-based independent research charity), http://genome.wellcome.ac.uk/doc _WTD020948.html, accessed September 22, 2005.

5. BBC, "Historic Figures, James Lind (1716–1794)," http://www.bbc.co .uk/history/historic_figures/lind_james.shtml, accessed May 6, 2008.

6. John P. Swann, "History of the FDA," FDA History Office (adapted from George Kurian, ed., *A Historical Guide to the U.S. Government* [New York: Oxford University Press, 1998]), http://www.fda.gov/oc/history/historyoffda/default.htm, accessed May 6, 2008.

7. Donna Hamilton, "A Brief History of the Center for Drug Evaluation and Research," FDA History Office, November 1997, http://www .fda.gov/cder/about/history/Histext.htm, accessed May 6, 2008.

8. "Milestones in U.S. Food and Drug Law History," FDA Backgrounder, May 3, 1999, updated August 2005, http://www.fda.gov/opacom/backgrounders/miles.html, accessed March 18, 2008.

9. Appelbaum interview.

10. National Cancer Institute, U.S. National Institutes of Health, "What Is Randomization?" http://www.cancer.gov/clinicaltrials/understanding/what-is-randomization, accessed May 9, 2008.

11. Carol Ballantine, "Taste of Raspberries, Taste of Death—The 1937 Elixir Sulfanilamide Incident," *U.S. Food and Drug Administration Consumer Magazine*, June 1981, http://www.fda.gov/oc/history/elixir.html, accessed March 18, 2008.

12. Ibid.

13. "A Brief History of the Center for Drug Evaluation and Research," http://www.fda.gov/cder/about/history/page21.htm, accessed May 8, 2008.

14. Carol K. Redmond, John Stephenson, and Theodore Colton, *Biostatistics in Clinical Trials* (New York: John Wiley and Sons, 2001), 239.

15. "Medical Experiments of the Holocaust and Nazi Medicine," http://www.remember.org/educate/medexp.html, accessed May 8, 2008.

16. Redmond, Stephenson, et al., 239.

17. Robert Jay Lifton, *The Nazi Doctors: Medical Killing and the Psychology of Genocide* (New York: Basic Books, 2000), 337–83.

18. Author interview with Ken Faulkner, March 19, 2007.

19. Evelyne Shuster, "Fifty Years Later: The Significance of the Nuremberg Code," *New England Journal of Medicine*, 337, no. 20 (November 13, 1997): 1436–40.

20. Division of Research and Graduate Studies, Office for the Protection of Research Subjects, University of Nevada at Las Vegas, "History of Research Ethics," http://research.unlv.edu/OPRS/history-ethics.htm, accessed May 8, 2008

21. Shuster, 1439.

22. Donna Hamilton, "A Brief History of the Center for Drug Evaluation and Research," FDA History Office, November 1997, http://www.fda.gov/CDER/about/history/Histext.htm, accessed July 14, 2008.

23. Appelbaum interview.

24. Baruch C. Cohen, "The Ethics of Using Medical Data from Nazi Experiments," *Jewish Law*, August 2006, 11, http://www.jlaw.com/Articles/NaziMedEx.html, accessed March 18, 2008.

25. Ibid., 17.

26. Ibid., 14–17.

27. Ibid., 2.

28. U.S. Department of Health and Human Services, Centers for Disease Control and Prevention, "U.S. Public Health Service Syphilis Study at Tuskegee," *The Tuskegee Timeline, The Study Begins,* January 9, 2008, http://www.cdc.gov/tuskegee/timeline.htm, accessed May 9, 2008.

29. Ibid.

30. James H. Jones, *Bad Blood: The Tuskegee Syphilis Experiment* (New York: Free Press, 1981), 4.

31. Ibid.

32. U.S. Department of Health and Human Services, U.S. Public Health Study.

33. UNLV, "History of Research Ethics."

34. World Medical Association Helsinki Declaration, adopted by the 18th World Medical Assembly, Helsinki, Finland, June 1964. Amended by the 29th World Medical Assembly, Tokyo, Japan, October 1975; 35th

World Medical Assembly, Venice, Italy, October 1983; and the 41st World Medical Assembly, Hong Kong, September 1989, Basic Principals.

35. Jones, 11.

36. Pearson Education, "The Tuskegee Syphilis Experiment," Information Please Database, Inc., 2007, http://www.infoplease.com/ipa/A0762136.html, accessed May 9, 2008.

37. Ibid.

38. Associated Press, "Tuskegee Syphilis Study's Fallout Debated: Researchers Split Over Whether Blacks Are More Mistrustful of Clinical Trials," March 16, 2008, http://www.msnbc.msn.com/id/23659667/, accessed July 14, 2008.

39. Appelbaum interview.

40. Amanda Gardner, "Black Americans Still Wary of Clinical Trials," *US News & World Report,* January 14, 2008, http://health.usnews.com/usnews/health/healthday/080114/black-americans-still-wary-of-clinical-trials.htm, accessed July 14, 2008.

41. Associated Press, "Tuskegee Syphilis Study's Fallout Debated."

42. "An Apology 65 Years Late," *NewsHour with Jim Lehrer* program transcript, May 16, 1997, http://www.pbs.org/newshour/bb/health/may97/tuskegee_5-16a.html, accessed July 14, 2008.

43. Larry M. Grant, Patricia A. Stewart, and Vincent J. Lynch, *Social Workers Speak Out on the HIV/AIDS Crisis* (Westport, CT: Greenwood Publishing Group, 1998), 9.

44. Jonathan Engel, *The Epidemic: A Global History of AIDS* (New York: HarperCollins, 2006), 287.

45. Faulkner interview.

46. Jonathan D. Moreno, *Undue Risk: Secret State Experiments on Humans* (New York: Routledge, 2000), 249.

47. Jordan Goodman, Anthony McElligott, and Lara Marks, eds., *Useful Bodies: Humans in the Service of Medical Science in the Twentieth Century* (Baltimore: JHU Press, 2003), 127.

48. Appelbaum interview.

49. "Whatever Happened to Polio?" Smithsonian National Museum of American History, http://americanhistory.si.edu/polio/virusvaccine/clinical.htm, accessed May 9, 2008.

50. Ibid.

51. Sonia Shah, *The Body Hunters* (New York and London: The New Press, 2006), 4.

52. Jonathan R. Carapetis, book review of *The Cutter Incident: How America's First Polio Vaccine Led to the Growing Vaccine Crisis*, by Paul A. Offit, M.D., *BMJ* magazine, March 26, 2006, 733.

53. Faulkner interview.

54. Author interview with Alan Milstein, January 31, 2008.

55. "From Test Tube to Patient: Protecting America's Health Through Human Drugs," *FDA Consumer Magazine* and the FDA Center for Drug Evaluation and Research, fourth edition, January 2006, http://www.fda.gov/fdac/special/testtubetopatient/default.htm, accessed July 14, 2008.

56. CNN, staff and wire reports, "FDA Suspends Trials at Gene Therapy Lab," January 22, 2000, http://archives.cnn.com/2000/HEALTH/01/22/gene.therapy/index.html, accessed March 18, 2008.

57. Emily Sanders, "AAMC Announces New Set of Rules for Medical Researchers," *Daily Pennsylvanian*, January 9, 2002, 1.

58. CNN, staff and wire reports, "FDA Suspends Trials at Gene Therapy Lab."

59. Sheryl Gay Stolberg, "Teenager's Death Is Shaking Up Field of Human Gene-Therapy Experiments," *New York Times*, January 27, 2000, http://query.nytimes.com/gst/fullpage.html?res=990CE6DC123CF934A15752C0A9669C8B63&sec=&spon=&pagewanted=1, accessed March 18, 2008.

60. Sheryl Gay Stolberg, "Senators Press For Answers On Gene Trials," *New York Times*, February 3, 2000, http://query.nytimes.com/gst/fullpage.html?res=9502E1DD133FF930A35751C0A9669C8B63, accessed March 1, 2008.

61. Robert J. Derocher, "Healthcare Gamble," *Insight* (a publication of the Illinois chapter of the Certified Public Accountant Society), April/May 2003, 34–37.

62. Ibid.

63. "Research Halt," *NewsHour with Jim Lehrer* program transcript, July 20, 2001, http://www.pbs.org/newshour/bb/health/july-dec01/hopkins_7-20.html, accessed March 18, 2008.

64. Scott Graham, "Johns Hopkins Leads Changes in Human Studies Process," *Baltimore Business Journal*, July 22, 2002, http://bizjournals .com/baltimore/stories/2002/07/22/focus1.html.

65. Derocher.

66. Ibid.

67. *Publishers Weekly*, May 2, 2006, http://www.amazon.ca/Great-Starvation-Experiment-Starved-Millions/dp/0743270304, accessed July 14, 2008.

68. "FDA Approves Gleevec for Pediatric Leukemia Treatment," *FDA News*, May 20, 2003, http://fda.gov/bbs/topic/news/2003/new00909 .html.

69. George J. Annas and Sherman Elias, "Thalidomide and the Titanic: Reconstructing the Technology Tragedies of the Twentieth Century," *American Journal of Public Health* 89, no. 1 (January 1998): 98–102.

70. Ibid.

71. Appelbaum interview.

72. "Vioxx (rofecoxib) Questions and Answers," prepared by the FDA, September 30, 2004, http://www.fda.gov/CDER/DRUG/infopage/ vioxx/vioxxQA, accessed May 11, 2008.

73. Snigdha Prakash and Vikki Valentine, "Timeline: The Rise and Fall of Vioxx," National Public Radio, June 8, 2006, http://www.npr.org/ templates/story/story.php?storyId=5470430, accessed July 14, 2008.

74. Ibid.

75. Eric J. Topol, "Failing the Public Health—Rofecoxib, Merck, and the FDA," *New England Journal of Medicine* 351, no. 17 (October 21, 2004): 1707–9.

76. Ibid.

77. Shelley Wood, "Dr. Eric Topol Denies Conflict of Interest Over Vioxx Condemnation," *MedScape Today*, from WebMD, December 3, 2004, http://www.medscape.com/viewarticle/538035, accessed May 11, 2008.

78. Author interview with Vera Sharav, March 1, 2007.

79. Faulkner interview.

80. Applebaum interview.

81. Ibid.

82. Author interview with Dr. Ezekiel Emanuel, January 2, 2008.

83. Gina Kolata, "Diabetes Study Verifies Lifesaving Tactic," *New York Times*, December 22, 2005, http://www.nytimes.com/2005/12/22/health/22diabetes.html, accessed March 18, 2008.

84. Ibid.

85. Gina Kolata, "Diabetes Study Partially Halted After Deaths," *New York Times*, February 7, 2008, http://www.nytimes.com/2008/02/07/health/07diabetes.html?_r=1&scp=2&sq=diabetes&st=nyt&oref=login, accessed March 18, 2008.

86. Kolata, "Diabetes Study Verifies Lifesaving Tactic."

87. Kolata, "Diabetes Study Halted After Deaths."

88. Ibid.

89. Ibid.

90. Multi-state Lottery Association, "Powerball Odds and Chances, 1997–2007," http://www.winningwithnumbers.com/lottery/games/powerball/, accessed July 14, 2008.

91. Faulkner interview.

Chapter 3: MONEY MAKES THE TRIAL GO 'ROUND

1. Author interview with Dr. David Satin, October 18, 2007.

2. BCC Research, "Report Highlights," *The Clinical Trials Business*, August 1, 2006, http://www.bccresearch.com/Report/PHM027B.html, accessed July 14, 2008.

3. Author interview with Doug Peddicord, executive director Association of Clinical Research Organizations, January 9, 2008.

4. Peddicord interview.

5. Sameer S. Chopra, "Industry Funding of Clinical Trials: Benefit or Bust?" *Journal of the American Medical Association*, July 2, 2003, 113, http://jama.ama-assn.org/cgi/reprint/290/1/113.pdf, accessed July 14, 2008.

6. Peter E. Carlson, "Clinical Research Industry Trends," National Center on Education and the Economy report (January 2007): 1.

7. Carl Elliott, "Guinea Pigging: Healthy human subjects for drug-safety trials are in demand. But is it a living?" *New Yorker*, January 7, 2008, 37.

8. Bill Alpert, "The State of Statins," *Barron's*, June 14, 2004, http://www

.smartmoney.com/barrons/index.cfm?story=20040614, accessed January 30, 2007.

9. Author interview with James McKenney, president and CEO, National Clinical Research, March 16, 2007.

10. The Center for Information & Study on Clinical Research Participation (CISCRP), "Facts & Figures," http://www.ciscrp.org/information/facts.asp, accessed January 29, 2007.

11. Ibid., 3.

12. Carlson, 1.

13. Milt Freudenheim, "Showdown Looms in Congress Over Drug Advertising on TV," *New York Times*, January 22, 2007, http://www.nytimes.com/2007/01/22/business/media/22drug.html?ref=washington, accessed July 14, 2008.

14. Geeta Anand, "Lab Rat?" *Wall Street Journal*, December 15, 2007.

15. Ibid., 2.

16. Ibid.

17. Thomas Goetz, "Practicing Patients," *New York Times Magazine*, March 23, 2008, http://www.nytimes.com/2008/03/23/magazine/23patients-t.html?pagewanted=1&_r=1&hp, accessed May 17, 2008.

18. Anand.

19. Ibid.

20. Jamie Talan, "Parkinson's Patients Want Experimental Drug on Market," *Newsday*, November 21, 2004, http://www.parkinsons-information-exchange-network-online.com/parkmail1/2004d/msg00670.html, accessed July 14, 2008.

21. Ibid.

22. Andrew Pollack, "Patients in Test Won't get Drug, Amgen Decides," *New York Times*, February 15, 2005.

23. Ibid.

24. Carlson, 2.

25. Transcript of advertisement; video provided by Clinical Trial Media, Inc., to author on July 25, 2007.

26. George J. Annas, "Questing for Grails: Duplicity, Betrayal, and Self-Deception in Post-Modern Medical Research," in *Health and Human Rights, A Reader*, edited by Jonathan Mann, Sofia Gruskin, Michael A. Grodin, and George J. Annas (New York: Routledge, 1999), 326.

27. Ibid.

28. "Advisory Committee on Human Radiation Experiments," *Final Report* (New York: Oxford University Press, 1996), 734.

29. Annas, 324.

30. Ibid.

31. Carol Rados, "Truth in Advertising: Rx Drugs Come of Age," *FDA Consumer Magazine*, July–August 2004, http://www.fda.gov/fdac/features/2004/404_ads.html, accessed July 14, 2008.

32. Ibid.

33. Stephanie Saul, "Pfizer to End Lipitor Campaign by Jarvik," *New York Times*, February 25, 2008, http://www.nytimes.com/2008/02/25/business/25cnd-pfizer.html?em&ex=1204088400&en=bef5d1b2511bbb64%0A, accessed July 14, 2008.

34. Clinical Trial Media, Inc. Web site, http://www.clinicaltrialmedia.com/index_true.htm, accessed February 3, 2008.

35. Business report on Clinical Trial Media, Inc., posted by Manta, February 3, 2008, accessed at http://www.manta.com/coms2/dnbcompany_dfm1zw.

36. MMG home page, http://www.mmgct.com/mmg/, accessed February 4, 2008.

37. Diversified Agency Services search for companies in specialty areas, http://www.dasglobal.com/results.lasso, accessed February 4, 2008.

38. Omnicom Group, Inc., company profile, Yahoo! Finance, http://biz.yahoo.com/ic/14/14326.html, accessed February 4, 2008.

39. Centralized Recruitment Advertising, report, Clinical Trial Media, Inc., July 23, 2007.

40. McKenney interview.

41. Frost and Sullivan, "CRO Industry at a Glance," Association of Clinical Research Organizations Web site, http://www.acrohealth.org/industry-ataglance.php, accessed February 4, 2008.

42. Frost and Sullivan, CenterWatch estimates, *World Contract Research Organizations Markets*, http://www.acrohealth.org/industry-ataglance.php, accessed February 4, 2008.

43. Peddicord interview.

44. McKenney interview.

45. Ibid.

46. Author interview with Joe Giffels, February 4, 2009.

47. McKenney interview.

48. "A Drug's Journey to Failure" (graphic accompanying the article "End of Drug Trial Is a Big Loss for Pfizer"), *New York Times*, December 3, 2006.

49. Sam Lister, "Drug Trial Axed After Patients Poisoned," *The Times Online*, March 15, 2006, http://www.timesonline.co.uk/tol/news/uk/article741160.ece, accessed October 14, 2008.

50. Elisabeth Rosenthal, "When Drug Trials Go Horribly Wrong," *International Herald Tribune*, April 9, 2006.

51. Miriam Shuchman, "Commercializing Clinical Trials—Risks and Benefits of the CRO Boom," *New England Journal of Medicine* 357, no. 14 (October 7, 2007): 1365–68.

52. Ibid.

53. Ibid., 1368.

54. Ibid., 1367.

55. Douglas Peddicord, "ACRO Responds on CROs and the Clinical Research Enterprise," October 12, 2007, http://www.acrohealth.org/highlight-detail.php?serial=32, accessed May 29, 2008.

56. "CRO Industry in FDA Limbo? NEJM Indicts CROs," October 18, 2007, http://www.clinpage.com/article/nejm_indicts_cros/C15, accessed May 30, 2008.

57. Thomas Bodenheimer, "Uneasy Alliance—Clinical Investigators and the Pharmaceutical Industry," *New England Journal of Medicine* 342, no. 20 (May 18, 2000): 1539–44.

58. John Carroll, "Crowing About Their Growth," *Biotechnology Healthcare*, December 2005, 47.

59. Bodenheimer, 2.

60. Peddicord interview.

61. Author interview with Ezekiel J. Emanuel, January 2, 2008.

62. "Understanding Clinical Trials," FDA, http://www.clinicaltrials.gov/ct2/info/understand, accessed February 16, 2007.

63. Bodenheimer, 2.

64. Ibid.

65. Ibid.

66. Ibid., 3.

67. Ibid.

68. Benedict Carey, "Antidepressant Studies Unpublished," *New York Times*, January 17, 2008.

69. Alex Berenson, "Accusation of Delays in Releasing Drug Results," *New York Times*, April 1, 2008.

70. Ibid.

71. Ibid.

72. Author interview with Dr. Harlan Krumholz, May 21, 2008.

73. Carey.

74. Krumholz interview.

75. Bodenheimer, 4.

76. Krumholz interview.

77. Chopra.

78. "Sponsorship, Authorship, and Accountability," editorial, *New England Journal of Medicine* 345, no. 11 (September 13, 2001): 825–27.

79. Job listings for "clinical research organizations" posted on Jobster.com, http://www.jobster.com/find/US/jobs/for/clinical+research+organizations, accessed February 19, 2008.

80. *American Way*, February 1, 2008, 52.

81. *Applied Clinical Trials*, December 1, 2007, http://actmagazine.findpharma.com/appliedclinicaltrials/article/articleDetail.jsp?id=477827&pageID=1&sk=&date=, accessed February 19, 2008.

82. Association of American Medical Colleges listing of Clinical Research Training Programs, updated July 11, 2007, http://www.aamc.org/research/clinicalresearch/training/start.htm, accessed February 19, 2008.

83. Sabine Vollmer, "Do You Know Science? Drug Companies Want You," *News & Observer*, October 20, 2007, D1.

84. Author interview with Melissa Ockert, February 19, 2008.

85. WRAL News, "With $25 Million in Incentives, Quintiles Decides to Stay in Durham, Plans to Add 1,000 Jobs," November 30, 2006.

86. Sabine Vollmer, "INC to Add 1,100 Jobs, May Get $14.8 Million," *News & Observer*, October 11, 2007, D1.

87. Ibid.

88. Jon Thompson, Patricia Baird, and Jocelyn Downie, *The Olivieri Report: The Complete Text of the Report of the Independent Inquiry*

Commissioned by the Canadian Association of University Teachers (Halifax, NS: Lorimer, 2001), 5.

89. Ibid., 7

90. Ibid., 9–10.

91. Jon Thompson, Patricia A. Baird, and Jocelyn Downie, "The Olivieri Case: Context and Significance," *Ecclectica*, December 2005, http://www.ecclectica.ca/issues/2005/3/index.asp?Article=2, accessed February 20, 2008.

92. C. K. Gunsalus, Edward M. Bruner, Nicholas C. Burbules, Leon Dash, Matthew Finkin, Joseph P. Goldberg, William T. Greenough, Gregory A. Miller, and Michael G. Pratt, "Mission Creep in the IRB World," editorial, *Science*, 312, no. 5779 (2006): 1441.

93. Ibid.

94. Author interview with Susie Hoffman, RN, BSN, CIP, director, Human Investigation Committee, University of Virginia, March 30, 2007.

95. Gunsalus, Bruner, et al.

96. Ibid.

97. Ibid.

98. Jill Wechsler, "FDA Hit for Poor Clinical Trial Oversight," *Applied Clinical Trials*, November 1, 2007, http://actmagazine.findpharma.com/appliedclinicaltrials/View+from+Washington/FDA-Hit-for-Poor-Clinical-Trial-Oversight/ArticleStandard/Article/detail/468088?contextCategoryId=553, accessed February 20, 2008.

Chapter 4: LEGAL TRIALS

1. Sheryl Gay Stolberg, "On Medicine's Frontier: The Last Journey of James Quinn," *New York Times*, October 8, 2002, http://www.sskrplaw.com/publications/021008.html, accessed March 5, 2008.

2. Stacey Burling, "Life, but at What Cost? The Inside Story of Artificial Heart Pioneer James "Butch" Quinn—an Emotional Odyssey Where Good Intentions, Hopes and Dreams Weren't," *Philadelphia Inquirer*, September 29, 2002, http://www.sskrplaw.com/publications/020929.html, accessed March 4, 2008.

3. Author interview with Alan Milstein, January 31, 2008.

4. Stolberg.

5. Ibid.

6. Burling.

7. Stolberg.

8. Ibid.

9. Burling.

10. Dr. Douglas R. Mackintosh, "Does Litigation Raise Standards of Care in Clinical Research? Healthy Hunting? Why the 'Junkyard Dog' Is a Necessary Protection," *Good Clinical Practice Journal*, January 2003, 25–26.

11. Milstein interview.

12. Ibid.

13. Stolberg.

14. Quinn Complaint, filed in the Court of Common Pleas, Philadelphia County, October 2002, on behalf of Irene Quinn by Alan C. Milstein and Derek T. Braslow of the law firm Sherman, Silverstein, Kohl, Rose & Podolsky.

15. Maureen Milford, "Lawsuits Attack Medical Trials[,] As claims arise, some fear tests will lose public support," *National Law Journal* (August 20, 2001), http://sskrplaw.com/publications/medicaltrials.html.

16. Ibid.

17. Ibid.

18. Vida Foubister, "Clinical trial patients sue IRB members[,] Suit could hinder medical research if individual institutional review board members are found liable," *American Medical News*, February 26, 2001, http://www.ama-assn.org/amednews/2001/02/26/prsb0226.htm, accessed July 14, 2008.

19. Ibid.

20. Jennifer Washburn, "Informed Consent—Alan Milstein says he wants to rescue us from unscrupulous doctors, undisclosed risks and greedy institutions. But is he a shining knight, or an enemy of medical progress?" *Washington Post Magazine*, December 30, 2001, http://www.sskrplaw.com/publications/informed.html, accessed March 9, 2008.

21. Milford.

22. Ibid.

23. Milstein interview.

24. Sarah Rubenstein, "When Drug Trials Go Wrong, Patients Have

Little Recourse," *Wall Street Journal*, http://online.wsj.com/article/SB120173515260330205.html?mod=hpp_us_pageone, accessed March 9, 2008.

25. Ibid.

26. Ibid.

27. Ibid.

28. Carl Elliott, "Guinea-pigging: Healthy human subjects for drug-safety trials are in demand. But is it a living," *New Yorker*, January 7, 2008, 40.

29. "Rise in Litigation Claim Activity Prompts Self Analysis of Industry's Clinical Trials; Chubb, E&Y to Host Panel on Ethical Considerations at BIO Conference," *Business Wire*, June 25, 2001.

30. Washburn.

31. Milstein interview.

32. Washburn.

33. Ibid.

34. Milstein interview.

35. Mackintosh, 26.

36. Stephen DeCherney, "Does Litigation Raise Standards of Care in Clinical Research? Hunting the Wrong Quarry—Why the Market Works Best to Maintain GCP," *Good Clinical Practice Journal* (January 2003): 26–27.

37. Gardiner Harris and Alex Berenson, "Drug Makers Near Old Goal: A Legal Shield," *New York Times*, April 6, 2008, http://www.nytimes.com/2008/04/06/washington/06patch.html?_r=2&hp&oref=slogin&oref=slogin, accessed May 13, 2008.

38. David Stout, "Justices Make It Tougher to Sue Medical Device Makers," *New York Times*, February 20, 2008, http://www.nytimes.com/2008/02/20/washington/20cnd-device.html?hp, accessed May 13, 2008.

39. Milstein interview.

Chapter 5: THERE'S A SUBJECT BORN EVERY MINUTE

1. "MDS Pharma Services Expands Early Clinical Research Facility in Phoenix, Arizona," MDS Pharma Services news release distributed by PRNewswire via COMTEX, October 3, 2002.

2. MDS Web site, http://www.mdsinc.com/investors/index.asp and http://www.mdsps.com/Company/Default.aspx, January 19, 2008.

3. Author research, December 2007–January 2008.

4. MDS Pharma Services information packet for Study # AA42951_9, January 17, 2008, 5.

5. Ibid., 1.

6. Author research, January 17, 2008.

7. Ibid.

8. MDS Pharma Services Project No. AA42961 consent form, version 6.0, 4–5.

9. Ibid., 6.

10. Robert Helms, "The Guinea Pig Strike at PENN 1935," *Guinea Pig Zero: An Anthology of the Journal for Human Research Subjects* (New Orleans: Garrett County Press, 2002), 83.

11. W. Osler Abbott, "The Problems of the Professional Guinea Pig," *Proceedings of the Charaka Club, Volume 10*, 1941, 249–60.

12. Helms, 85.

13. Ibid., 86.

14. Carl Elliott, "Guinea Pigging: Healthy human subjects for drug-safety trials are in demand. But is it a living?" *New Yorker*, January 7, 2007, 36.

15. Ibid.

16. Barbara Solow, "The Secret Lives of Guinea Pigs: An edgy occupation moves into the mainstream as the local market for human test subjects booms," *Independent Weekly* (February 9, 2000): 3, www.indyweek.com, http://www.indyweek.com/gyrobase/Content?oid=13968, accessed March 12, 2008.

17. Elliott, 37.

18. Laurie P. Cohen, "Lilly's 'Quick Cash' to Habitués of Shelters Vanishes Quickly," *Wall Street Journal*, November 14, 1996, http://www.oralchelation.com/taheebo/foottah/lilly.htm, accessed March 10, 2008.

19. Ibid.

20. Ibid.

21. Ibid.

22. Ibid.

23. Ibid.

24. Ibid.

25. Ibid.

26. David Evans, Michael Smith, and Liz Wille, "Human Guinea Pigs Pay for Lax FDA Rules," *Bloomberg News* (published in the *Seattle Times*, November 6, 2005), http://seattletimes.nwsource.com/cgi-bin/Print Story.pl?document_id=2002606640&zsection_id=2002119995&slug=drugtesting06&date=20051106, accessed March 12, 2008.

27. Ibid.

28. Ibid.

29. Ibid.

30. Ibid.

31. "SFBC Independent Report Refutes Most Bloomberg Allegations," *South Florida Business Journal*, December 15, 2005, http://www.bizjournals.com/stories/2005/12/12/daily48.html.

32. Elliott, 37–38.

33. Gene Marcial, "Testing Times for SFBC International," *Business Week*, November 5, 2005, http://www.businessweek.com/investor/content/nov2005/pi20051118_3323_pi001.htm, accessed March 13, 2008

34. Author interview with Ken Getz, founder and chairman of the Center for Information & Study on Clinical Research Participation and senior research fellow at the Center for the Study of Drug Development at Tufts University, January 11, 2008.

35. Elliott, 34.

36. MDS Pharma Services information packet, 3.

37. Ibid., 2.

38. Author research, January 17, 2008.

39. Elliott, 36.

40. Rebecca Meisner, "Guinea Pig Gang," *Cleveland Scene*, March 22, 2006, http://www.clevescene.com/2006-03-22/news/guinea-pig-gang/1, accessed July 14, 2008.

41. Meisner.

42. Solow, 5–6.

43. Ibid., 3.

44. Author interview with William Hirschhorn, director Clinical Research Organization and Management graduate program at the College of Medicine at Drexel University, March 1, 2007.

45. Author interview with Paul Clough, February 26, 2007.

46. Paul Clough, Guinea Pigs Get Paid Web site, http://www.gpgp.net/tips.php, accessed March 17, 2008.

47. Clough interview.

48. Solow, 4–5.

49. Elliott, 38.

50. Ibid., 39.

51. Meisner.

52. Ibid.

53. Michael Kranish, "System for Protecting Humans in Research Faulted," *Boston Globe*, March 25, 2002, http://www.boston.com/dailyglobe2/084/nation/System_for_protecting_humans_in _research_faulted+.shtml, accessed July 14, 2008.

54. Ibid.

55. Ibid.

56. Elliott, 38.

57. Kranish.

58. Elliott, 38.

59. Ibid., 36.

60. Ibid., 37.

61. Mikita Brottman, "I Was a Brain Slave," Guinea Pig Zero Web site, http://www.guineapigzero.com/brainslave.html, accessed March 14, 2008.

62. Ibid.

63. Ibid.

64. Drug study subject, "22 Nights and 23 Days: Diary of #1J," Guinea Pig Zero Web site, http://www.guineapigzero.com/23days.html, October 2006, accessed March 8, 2008.

65. Elliott, 40.

66. Author interview with Robert Helms, March 8, 2007.

67. Ibid.

68. David Futrelle, "Let the dogs bark: The quite-possibly true story of a human guinea pig who bit the hand that drew his blood," *Salon*, July 14, 1997, http://www.salon.com/july97/media/media970714.html, accessed March 15, 2008.

69. Ibid.

70. Solow.

71. Ibid., 6.

72. Ibid.

73. Author interview with Alan Milstein, January 31, 2008.

Chapter 6: GOING GLOBAL

1. dgdresearch Web site, http://www.dgdresearch.com/about/, accessed April 6, 2008.

2. Merriam-Webster Dictionary (online), http://mw4.mw.com/dictionary/naive accessed April 6, 2008.

3. Gregory Lopes, "Drug Makers Look East for Testing," *Washington Times*, December 8, 2007.

4. Author interview with Kathy Mayle, November 11, 2007.

5. Lopes.

6. "U.S. Drug Makers Turn to India, China for Testing," *Economic Times*, December 13, 2007, http://economictimes.indiatimes.com/News/News_By_Industry/Healthcare_Biotech/US_drug_makers_turn_to_India_China_for_testing/articleshow/2618885.cms, accessed April 7, 2008.

7. A. T. Kearney, "Make Your Move: Taking Clinical Trials to the Best Location," *Executive Agenda*, January 3, 2007, 60.

8. Kirsty Barnes, "Balancing the Clinical Scales," DrugResearcher.com, March 28, 2006, http://www.drugresearcher.com/news/ng.asp?n=66213-cutting-edge-information-india-clinical-trials-costs-patient-recruitment, accessed April 7, 2008.

9. Ibid.

10. U.S. Department of Health and Human Services; Food and Drug Administration; Center for Drug Evaluation and Research (CDER); Center for Biologics Evaluation and Research (CBER); Center for Devices and Radiological Health (CDRH), "Guidance for Industry[,] Acceptance of Foreign Clinical Studies," March 2001, 1.

11. Department of Health and Human Services Office of Inspector General, "The Globalization of Clinical Trials[,] A Growing Challenge in Protecting Human Subjects," September 2001, ii.

12. Finnuala Kelleher, "The Pharmaceutical Industry's Responsibility

for Protecting Human Subjects of Clinical Trials in Developing Nations," *Columbia Journal of Law and Social Problems* 38, no. 1 (October 19, 2004): 85.

13. Kelleher, 86.

14. Joe Stephens, "Testing Tidal Wave Hits Overseas; On Distant Shores, Drug Firms Avoid Delays and Scrutiny Series: The Body Hunters: Overwhelming the Watchdogs," *Washington Post*, December 18, 2000.

15. Kearney.

16. Ibid.

17. Gina Kolata, "Companies Facing Ethical Issue as Drugs Are Tested Overseas," *New York Times*, March 5, 2004, http://query.nytimes.com/gst/fullpage.html?res=9B02EFD7103FF936A35750C0A9629C8B63&sec=&spon=&pagewanted=2, accessed April 7, 2008.

18. Ibid.

19. Ibid.

20. Mayle interview.

21. Kolata.

22. Jennifer Kahn, "A Nation of Guinea Pigs," *Wired*, March, 2006, 1, http://www.wired.com/wired/archive/14.03/indiadrug.html?pg=2&topic=indiadrug&topic_set=, accessed April 9, 2008.

23. Kearney, 61.

24. Ibid.

25. Ibid., 4.

26. Kahn.

27. Author interview with Sandhya Srinivasan, April 17, 2008.

28. Kearney, 58.

29. Ibid., 60-61.

30. Ibid., 59-60.

31. Ibid., 58-59.

32. Mike Oboh, "Pfizer Faces $8.5 Billion Suit Over Nigeria Drug Trial," Reuters, September 30, 2007, http://www.reuters.com/article/newsOne/idUSL287662420070930?pageNumber=1&virtualBrandChannel=0, accessed April 12, 2008.

33. Joe Stephens, "Pfizer Faces Criminal Charges in Nigeria," *Washington Post*, May 30, 2007.

34. Ibid.

35. Ibid.

36. Ibid.

37. Author interview with Dr. Ben Faneye, April 17, 2008.

38. Ibid.

39. BBC News, "Drug Trials Outsourced to India," broadcast April 27, 2006, on BBC Two, http://news.bbc.co.uk/2/hi/south_asia/4932188.stm, accessed April 14, 2008.

40. Ibid.

41. Ibid.

42. Kahn.

43. Edward J. Mills and Sonal Singh, "Health, Human Rights, and the Conduct of Clinical Research Within Oppressed Populations," *Globalization and Health*, November 27, 2007, http://www.globalizationandhealth.com/content/3/1/10#B20, accessed April 14, 2008.

44. Sonal Singh, Khagendra Dahal, and Edward Mills, "Nepal's War on Human Rights: A Summit Higher Than Everest," *International Journal for Equity in Health*, June 28, 2005, http://www.equityhealthj.com/content/4/1/9, accessed April 14, 2008.

45. Ibid.

46. Sonia Shah, "Globalizing Clinical Research," *Nation*, June 13, 2002, 3, http://www.thenation.com/doc/20020701/shah/3, accessed April 14, 2008.

47. Peter Lurie and Sidney M. Wolfe, "Unethical Trials of Interventions to Reduce Perinatal Transmission of the Human Immunodeficiency Virus in Developing Countries," *New England Journal of Medicine* 337, no. 12 (September 18, 1997): 853–56.

48. Ibid.

49. Shah, 2.

50. Author interview with Dr. Peter Lurie, April 15, 2008.

51. Shah, 2.

52. Amy L. Fairchild and Ronald Bayer, "Uses and Abuses of Tuskegee," *Science*, May 1999, 919–20.

53. Lurie interview.

54. Ibid.

55. Ibid.

56. Introduction to the "World Medical Association Declaration of Helsinki Ethical Principles for Medical Research Involving Human Subjects Adopted by the 18th WMA General Assembly, Helsinki, Finland, June 1964, and amended by the 29th WMA General Assembly, Tokyo, Japan, October 1975; 35th WMA General Assembly, Venice, Italy, October 1983; 41st WMA General Assembly, Hong Kong, September 1989; 48th WMA General Assembly, Somerset West, Republic of South Africa, October 1996; and the 52nd WMA General Assembly, Edinburgh, Scotland, October 2000; Note of Clarification on Paragraph 29 added by the WMA General Assembly, Washington 2002, Note of Clarification on Paragraph 30 added by the WMA General Assembly, Tokyo 2004."

57. Philip J. Hilts, *Protecting America's Health: The FDA, Business, and 100 Years of Regulation* (New York: Alfred A. Knopf, 2003), 225.

58. Tom Hollon, "FDA Uneasy About Placebo Revision," *Nature Medicine* 7, no. 1 (2001): 7.

59. Vicki Brower, "Science versus ethics: new ethical guidelines regarding the use of placebos in clinical trials have sharpened the conflict between public health and patients' rights," *EMBO Reports* (European Molecular Biology Association) 2, no. 5 (2001): 365–66.

60. Ibid., 366.

61. Ibid.

62. Ibid.

63. Mary Pat Flaherty and Joe Stephens, "Pa. Firm Asks FDA to Back Experiment Forbidden in the U.S.," *Washington Post*, February 23, 2001.

64. Ibid.

65. Brower, 366.

66. Public Citizen Health Research Group, "Placebo-Controlled Drug Trial in Latin America Redesigned[;] Company Will Provide Active Treatment to All Infants," news release, April 4, 2001, http://www.citizen.org/pressroom/release.cfm?ID=607.

67. Kolata.

68. Mayle interview.

69. Kolata.

70. Robert Hinkley, "How Corporate Law Inhibits Social Responsibility,"

Business Ethics: Corporate Social Responsibility Report, January/February 2002, 1.

71. Ibid.

72. Ibid.

73. Author interview with Dr. Ezekiel Emanuel, January 2, 2008.

74. Sonia Shah, *The Body Hunters* (New York: The New Press, 2006), 176.

75. Ibid., 175–76.

76. Lurie interview.

77. Bill HR 5249, "Safe Overseas Human Testing Act," 107th Congress, 2d Session, "To promote safe and ethical clinical trials of drugs and other test articles on people overseas," introduced in the U.S. House of Representatives, July 26, 2002, 1.

78. Ibid., 2–3.

79. Joe Stephens and Mary Pat Flaherty, "Regulation of Overseas Drug Trials Is Pursued, Legislation Limits Risky Medical Tests," *Washington Post*, August 4, 2001.

80. Ibid.

81. GovTrack.us, "H.R. 5641 [109th]: Safe Overseas Human Testing Act," http://www.govtrack.us/congress/bill.xpd?bill=h109-5641, accessed April 23, 2008.

82. Faneye interview.

Chapter 7: THE PERFECT LABORATORY
FOR CLINICAL TRIALS

1. Government of Uganda, UNGASS (United Nations General Assembly Special Session declaration of commitment on HIV and AIDS) Country Progress Report, Uganda, January 2006–December 2007, January 2008, 1.

2. AVERT, AVERTing HIV and AIDS, an International AIDS Charity, "The History of AIDS in Uganda," http://www.avert.org/aidsuganda.htm, accessed July 3, 2008.

3. "HIV/AIDS Surveillance Report: Cases of HIV Infection and AIDS in the United States and Dependent Areas, 2006," Basic statistics,

Centers for Disease Control and Prevention, May 22, 2008, http://www.cdc.gov/hiv/topics/surveillance/basic.htm#hivest, accessed July 12, 2008.

4. UNGASS Report, 2.

5. AVERT.

6. W. L. Kirungi, J. B. Musinguzi, A. Opio, and E. Madraa, "Trends in HIV prevalence and sexual behaviour (1990–2000) in Uganda," presented at the International Conference on AIDS, 2002, http://gateway.nlm.nih.gov/MeetingAbstracts/ma?f=102253576.html, accessed July 3, 2008.

7. Author interview with Father John Mary Mooka, June 15, 2008.

8. Francis Weyzig and Irene Schipper and SOMO (Centre for Research on Multinational Corporations), "Nevirapine PMTCT Trials in Uganda," SOMO briefing paper on ethics in clinical trials, 4, http://www.wemos.nl/Documents/clinical_%20trials_%20report.pdf, accessed July 12, 2008.

9. Gus Cairnes, "CROI: Microbicide Failure Poses More Questions Than Answers," *AIDS Map News*, February 28, 2007, http://www.aidsmap.com/en/news/678AA203-320E-42B6-9114-4F323CED09D8.asp, accessed July 10, 2008.

10. Father John Mary Mooka Kamweri, " 'Do No Harm': An Ethical Analysis of the Failed Microbicide Gel Clinical Trial in Uganda," April 20, 2008, 3.

11. PlusNews, "South Africa: When a microbicide trial goes wrong—Part 1," PlusNews Global HIV/AIDS news and analysis, October 9, 2007, http://www.plusnews.org/Report.aspx?ReportId=74717, accessed July 10, 2008.

12. Moses Paul Sserwanga, "Uganda Needs Law on Trial Medicines, October 16, 2007, http://msserwanga.blogspot.com/2007/10/uganda-needs-law-on-trial-medicines.html, accessed July 10, 2008.

13. Ibid.

14. Author interview with Dr. Pontiano Kaleebu, June 4, 2008.

15. Author interview with Peter Ssamula Kiwanuka, June 4, 2008.

16. Kaleebu interview.

17. Ibid.

18. Ibid.

19. Author interview with Charles (last name withheld for confidentiality), June 8, 2008.

20. Ibid.

21. Ibid.

22. Author interview with Jackson (last name withheld for confidentiality), contemporaneously interpreted from Luganda to English by Dr. Dennis Bbaale, June 7, 2008.

23. Ibid.

24. Author interview with Rose (last name withheld for confidentiality), contemporaneously interpreted from Luganda to English by Dr. Dennis Bbaale, June 7, 2008.

25. Ibid.

26. Author interview with Annett (last name withheld for confidentiality), contemporaneously interpreted from Luganda to English by Dr. Dennis Bbaale, June 7, 2008.

27. Ibid.

28. Ibid.

29. Christopher Mason, "Delivering Health Care on U.S.$19 Per Capita," *CMAJ*, January 15, 2008, http://www.cmaj.ca/cgi/content/full/178/2/135#FB16, accessed July 7, 2008. Copyright 1995–2008, Canadian Medical Association. All rights reserved. ISSN 1488-2329 (e) 0820-3946 (p).

30. Author interview with Paul Simon Mayanja, June 4, 2008.

31. Ibid.

32. Ibid.

33. Ibid.

34. Author interview with Dr. Martin Nsubuga, June 5, 2008.

35. Ibid.

36. Ibid.

37. Ibid.

38. Author interview with Dr. Medi Kawuma, June 5, 2008.

39. Ibid.

40. Ibid.

41. Ibid.

42. Author interview with doctor at Nsambya Hospital whose name has been withheld for confidentiality, June 5, 2008.

43. Author interview with Prof. David Serwadda, June 6, 2008.

44. Ibid.

45. E-mail to the author from Gulden Mesara, a representative from Pfizer, Inc., May 8, 2008.

46. Jon A. Story and David Kritchevsky, "Biographical Article, Denis Parsons Burkitt (1911–1993)," *The Journal of Nutrition*, American Institute of Nutrition, April 20, 1994, 1551, http://jn.nutrition.org/cgi/reprint/124/9/1551.pdf, accessed July 12, 2008.

47. Author interview with Dr. John C. Ssali, June 10, 2008.

48. Ibid.

49. Ibid.

50. Ibid.

51. Ibid.

52. Kawuma interview.

53. Ibid.

Chapter 8: THE STORIES BEHIND THE SUBJECTS

1. Author interview with Chris, March 2, 2007.

2. Ibid.

3. Ibid.

4. "The psychology of clinical trials: understanding physician motivation and patient perception," Thompson Center Watch, Survey of 749 study volunteers, 2006, http://www.centerwatch.com/professional/cw_commentary_psychology.html.

5. Author interview with Mike, March 5, 2007.

6. Ibid.

7. Ibid.

8. Author interview with Dr. Paul Appelbaum, February 14, 2007.

9. Author interview with Dr. Ezekiel Emanuel, January 2, 2008.

10. Ibid.

11. Author interview with Sandra Burks, R.N., B.S.N., C.C.R.C., March 15, 2008.

12. Ibid.

13. Ibid.

14. Ibid.

15. Ibid.

16. Dominican Sisters St. Mary of the Spring, "Sr. Mary Andrew Matesich Dies at 66," news release, June 15, 2005, http://columbusdominicans .org/newsevents/pressreleases/press2005_3.htm.

17. Denise Grady, "Heeding a Call to Breast Cancer Treatments," *New York Times*, July 26, 2004.

18. Ibid.

19. Ibid.

20. News release from Dominican Sisters St. Mary of the Spring.

21. "The psychology of clinical trials," Thompson Center Watch.

22. Ibid., 3.

23. Author interview with doctor who wished to remain anonymous, October 2007.

24. Ibid.

25. Author interview with Lori Ratliff, RN, March 5, 2007.

26. Ibid.

27. Ibid.

28. Ibid.

29. University of Virginia, "U.Va. Doctors Perform Major Diabetes Procedure: First Islet Cell Transplant in Virginia," news release, June 14, 2004, http://www.healthsystem.virginia.edu/internet/news/Archives 04/islet-cell-transplant.cfm.

30. Ratliff interview.

31. Ibid.

32. Ibid.

33. Ibid.

34. CSL Behring, "Your Rights in a Clinical Trial," CSL Behring Web site, http://www.cslbehring.com/s1/cs/enco/1187378997566/con tent/1187378982333/content.htm, accessed April 29, 2008.

35. Emanuel interview.

36. Robert Finn, *Cancer Clinical Trials: Experimental Treatments & How They Can Help You* (O'Reilly & Associates, Inc., 1999), chapter 3.

37. CSL Behring, "Your Responsibilities," CSL Behring Web site,

http://www.cslbehring.com/s1/cs/enco/1187378997559/content/1187378982359/content.htm, accessed April 29, 2008.

38. Lindsay A. Hampson, Manish Agrawal, Steven Joffe, Cary P. Gross, Joel Verter, and Ezekiel J. Emanuel, "Patients' Views on Financial Conflicts of Interest in Cancer Research Trials," *New England Journal of Medicine* 335, no. 22 (November 30, 2006): 2330–37.

39. Ibid.

40. Associated Press, "Hospital Medical Research Boards Often Face Ethical Conflicts: Survey," November 29, 2006, http://www.cbc.ca/health/story/2006/11/29/research-conflicts.html, accessed April 29, 2008.

41. Ibid.

42. Hampson, Agrawal, et al., 2331.

43. Denise Grady, "Patient or Guinea Pig? Dilemma of Clinical Trials," *New York Times*, January 5, 1999, http://query.nytimes.com/gst/fullpage.html?res=9903E2DA173EF936A35752C0A96F958260&sec=health&pagewanted=print, accessed April 29, 2008.

44. Ibid.

45. Ibid.

46. Ibid.

47. Ibid.

48. Ibid.

49. Jerry Bowen, "Saving Amy," *48 Hours Mystery* (CBS), September 7, 2000.

50. Ellen Licking, "Gene Therapy: One Family's Story," *BusinessWeek*, July 12, 1999, at http://www.businessweek.com/1999/99_28/b3637001.htm, accessed April 30, 2008.

51. Bowen.

52. Licking.

53. Bowen.

54. CBS News, "Gene Therapy as a Treatment for Patients Who Suffer from Fanconi Anemia," January 1, 2001.

55. Author interview with Mary Ellen Eiler, April 30, 2008.

56. Ibid.

57. Ibid.

58. Author interview with Joe Giffels, February 4, 2008.

59. Ibid.

60. Ibid.

61. Ibid.

62. Ibid.

63. Author interview with Wendell Steele, March 7, 2007.

64. Ibid.

65. Ibid.

66. Author interview with Paul Gelsinger, February 14, 2008.

67. Ibid.

68. Ibid.

69. Paul Gelsinger, "Jesse's Intent," Citizens for Responsible Care and Research Web site, http://www.circare.org/submit/jintent.pdf, accessed May 2, 2008.

70. Ibid., 10.

71. Gelsinger interview.

72. Ibid.

73. Gelsinger, 11–12.

74. Gelsinger interview.

75. Gelsinger, 12.

76. Gelsinger interview.

77. Ibid.

78. Ibid.

79. Ibid.

80. Ibid.

81. Ibid.

Afterword: VOLUNTEERING FOR A CLINICAL TRIAL

1. Office for Human Subject Protection, University of Rochester Medical Center, "Volunteering for a Clinical Trial[,] Important Information You Need to Know," February 2003, http://www.urmc .rochester.edu/ohsp/volunteer_info.html, accessed May 15, 2008.

2. OHRP (Office for Human Research Protection), "Becoming a Research Volunteer[,] It's Your Decision," http://www.hhs.gov/ ohrp/outreach/documents/3panelfinal.pdf, accessed May 15, 2008.

3. Author interview with Paul Gelsinger, February 14, 2008.

INDEX

A NOTE ON THE AUTHOR

ALEX O'MEARA is a freelance journalist who has worked for the City News Bureau of Chicago, *Newsday*, the *Baltimore Sun* in Washington, D.C., KVOA, an NBC affiliate in Tucson, Arizona, and many other media organizations. Diagnosed with type 1 diabetes almost thirty years ago, he has completed several marathons. In an effort to cure his diabetes, he participated in a risky and groundbreaking clinical trial to receive a transplant of islet cells from several cadaver pancreases. This is his first book. He lives in Bisbee, Arizona.